Mark

Our Natural Diet

Healthy Body Publishing, United Kingdom
www.hbpublishing.com

A Healthy Body Publishing Book
0-9553800

Printed and bound by CPI Group (UK) Ltd, Croydon, CR0 4YY

First published in 2011 as a Healthy Body Publishing paperback
Hertfordshire, United Kingdom

ISBN: 978-0955380068

The Author

Mark Hines is an Exercise and Human Physiologist, and Biomechanist, currently living in Surrey, England. He is based at the British College of Osteopathic Medicine, where he lectures on physiology and research methods, and at the University of Roehampton, where he is a PhD researcher. He writes and teaches private courses on exercise, nutrition and the palaeolithic diet, and has written various books and articles on related subjects for a wide variety of readers. In his spare time he competes in the most demanding ultra-endurance adventure races in the world.

Disclaimer

This book was written to give information on diet, nutrition and health, and to discuss many of the misconceptions commonly expressed relating to these. The information contained is not to be taken as prescriptive and should not be interpreted as such, particularly in place of advice given on an individual basis by an appropriately qualified health-care professional.

Acknowledgements

I would like to thank my family and friends for all their support. I would particularly like to thank Dr. Simon Dyall for his friendship, advice, support and banter throughout the last few years. I also thank him for taking the time to read through the original manuscript of this book prior to publication, and for the recommendations that have been included as a result.

I thank all the people who read the draft manuscripts and contributed to the shaping of this edition: Tracy, Andre, Lisa, Stephen, Katy and Jane. I believe the book was made better for your feedback, and I appreciate all your recommendations. As ever, John Quinn has been a huge help as a reviewer and proofreader, and his help and friendship is deeply treasured. I also thank Phil Taylor for his help in proofreading.

Many of the topics discussed in this book were included due to misconceptions commonly passed between those interested in health, as relayed to me by people genuinely interested in improving their understanding, and who wanted to better inform others in accordance with the real evidence. I therefore thank all the people who have wanted to discuss such issues with me over recent years. Not everything could be included, because life is too short and the nincompoops too many, for there to be any worth in taking them all to account. Please accept this as my best effort for the time being, and future editions will expand the breadth of our crusade.

Dedication

Socrates said *"an honest man is always a child"*, and *"I am the wisest man alive, for I know one thing and that is that I know nothing."*

There are three fundamental aspects to human understanding: The ability to ask questions, an appreciation of how to interpret results and a preparedness, willingness, and fearlessness to change one's mind when presented with reliable evidence.

This book is dedicated to everyone who believes this to be true.

Contents

"They must find it difficult, those who have taken authority as truth, rather than truth as authority."

- Gerald Massey

Foreword

**"A scientific truth does not triumph by convincing its opponents
and making them see the light, but rather because its
opponents eventually die and a new generation grows up
that is familiar with it."**

- Max Planck

Our Natural Diet is a book I have wanted to write for more than a
decade. Initially I had tried to cobble some basic dietary
recommendations into a more general book on health and fitness, but
it quickly became apparent that something of greater depth was
required. My original studies in physiology were related to
adaptations through physical activity, but I had been equally
passionate about developing my understanding of nutrition and
biochemistry. Following completion of my undergraduate and
postgraduate degrees, I invested several years of research into
improving my understanding of human evolution, diet and health.
Perhaps curiously, this had been initiated as a means to develop my
understanding of biomechanics and physical therapy, but the
relationships between anatomical, physiological and nutritional
evolutionary adaptations are inextricably linked.

All animals adapt to be as efficient as possible at acquiring
their food. Hence, studying evolutionary adaptation for locomotion
incorporates the study of changes in the human gut, the brain, body
size, and changes in food procurement strategies, local ecologies and
other associated factors. It soon became apparent that much of the
information on dieting and nutrition missed the mark by some

i

considerable margin, at least partly because it seemed more focussed on creating the next 'new thing' rather than just a sensible, accurate and reasonable appraisal of the actual science of nutrition.

With this being the case I realised I ought to write two books on the subject. Although I had read much of Dr Loren Cordain's research when studying human evolution, his book, *The Paleo Diet*, seemed to require the reader to have too great an element of trust. Specifically, it included a statement referring to "work in my lab", which I resented a little. In a single book on diet the reader might well not be interested in all the research, and having read his research papers I happened to know he was being quite accurate, but still I disliked the idea the reader lacked the option to learn more about some of the topics. I would have liked references, details and evidence, and in that respect I felt there was a missed opportunity, and others might have felt likewise.

I wanted to write *Our Natural Diet* – or at least something with similar objectives to this book – but felt I needed to write another book first to explain the scientific background, so there would be absolutely no necessity for faith in the author. Readers could have all the important aspects of human evolution and diet explained, and have access to the titles of all the references included in the book (including Dr Cordain's original lab work). I accepted some people were unlikely to be interested in that level of background information, but I considered it a more appropriate step than to assume knowledge or deliver unsupported statements. Besides, it is my firm conviction that people typically *do* want the detail, because that deeper understanding generates far more interest than simple conclusions of "eat more of this and less of that."

The purpose of *Human Evolution, Diet and Health*, was to present the case for how an appreciation of our evolutionary heritage can be useful to better understand modern diets and nutrition. The

simple philosophy is that almost every aspect of our current biology –
including our digestive anatomy and all the physiological processes
associated with metabolism of foods – has changed little since
Palaeolithic times (the Old Stone Age). By understanding the gradual
adaptations to our diet and way of life, it becomes easy to see how our
decreased levels of physical activity and our over-consumption of
foods of convenience, have led to increases in overweightness, obesity
and many modern diseases. So, *Human Evolution, Diet and Health*
was intended to lay the groundwork, but was only ever meant to be an
informative text, rather than an instructional one.

The Palaeolithic diet is also only a model, there to help us
understand the challenges of living in a world we have lacked time to
adapt to, at least in the physiological sense. Palaeolithic foods,
including fruits, vegetables, meats and fish, do not exist now as they
did in our pasts. Agriculture and the food sciences have developed
foods selected and cultivated to match the needs of economies, land
resources, and changes in consumer tastes. The consequences of
modern industry include altered food and drink composition and
quality, with various sources of pollution finding their way into our
food chain. Although understanding our Palaeolithic heritage is
certainly useful for better understanding our own health and nutrition,
that model has to be viewed in the perspective of modern times, with
everything that comes with our current lifestyles, tastes and
conveniences.

Modern industries, an unnaturally focussed and consuming
work ethic, and a common will for convenience, has facilitated the
development of many problems now associated with life in
westernised societies. But science is coming of age, and technology is
now being positively used to improve food quality and better assess
risks and pollutants as they appear, with both local and worldwide
initiatives to promote health and limit disease.

Part of the message of this book is about accepting those aspects of modern living we can do little about, and finding ways to increase our intake of all the nutrients we need, whilst limiting total intakes of the substances with a potential to cause harm. It is down to the individual to decide whether the different aspects of our modern times are good, bad or inconsequential, but in all cases understanding the unique challenges of our times is useful for promoting our own good health. Whether we wish to alter our body weight or body composition is really only a matter of fine-tuning, using the basis of an optimally healthy diet as the most conducive starting point.

* * * * * * *

Our Natural Diet was written as much without prejudice and bias as was practically achievable. That is, what is actually included is not representative of the author's ideas when the project commenced. In order to write a book independent from *Human Evolution, Diet and Health*, it was important to conduct fresh reviews of the scientific literature related to diet and health, and in so doing new information came to light which had not been fully explored previously. What was going to be a page on toxins has become a full chapter, whereas the section on supplements has been greatly and necessarily condensed.

Although new research will add improved depth and understanding to the general points raised in this book, it is unlikely (although not impossible) any of the recommendations will have to be entirely re-worked. I would not be a scientist if I believed the information here could not be challenged, and it is natural that I should welcome this as an excuse for conducting further reviews of literature, as new studies emerge to challenge yesterday's research. As this occurs, so future editions will reflect this. In the interim, I will ensure relevant updates and amendments are included on my website (www.markhines.org).

*   *   *   *   *   *   *

Our Natural Diet is not a particularly catchy title. Whilst this is not an entirely deliberate feature, what is important is that the information and recommendations here are intended to be sensible, salient and reasonable. There is information to help inform choice, and recommendations based upon as good an evidence base as was available at the time of going to press. This is not a diet *per se*, but an approach. It is not supposed to be a new way of eating that begins tomorrow and lasts a fortnight. This book is about helping people to support their health and achieve whatever goals are reasonable within the confines of a good diet and healthy lifestyle.

The reality is that *Our Natural Diet* is so-called in preference to *The Natural Diet*, or, heaven forbid, *The Hines Diet* (I cringe at the very idea, even on the umpteenth edit of the draft). This is a book for anyone who wants to have a good understanding of the most recent research on nutrition, diet and health, a matter that should remain so as new chapters and articles are added via the website and any future editions. It is not for people who want to be told 'Eat this', 'Don't eat that'. It is for the intelligent, discerning individual, who can read between the lines and see this is a guide: 'More of these foods are good, and here is why you might want to consider ways of including more of them in your daily diet'; 'These foods are not as good as many people like to think, this is the science behind it, and if this seems reasonable to you then you might also want to substitute those foods with alternatives'. Take it or leave it, as I have nothing more to sell to you, and have no intention of devoting a lifetime in quibbles with everyone who writes an alternative. Besides, they might all be right.

I do like to think people are genuinely interested in the level of detail typically omitted or overlooked when it comes to health information. That detail is often of fundamental relevance when it comes to understanding the underlying physiology of how the body utilises or eliminates particular foods. To ensure as few stones as possible were left unturned, some of the chapters in this book do incorporate myriad examples from the related research, and perhaps go into the detail further than is absolutely required to support understanding. It is there, however, because some people do appreciate it and are keen to learn such things. For those less interested in these details it is perhaps better to skip through those areas, but keep in mind it is there should you ever wish to return to it at a later time.

This book is certainly not about pushing supplements on people who do not need them, and there had better not ever be a '*Natural Diet Recipe Book*', unless some leading chef wants to have a stab at it – it is beyond the scope of a researcher to write such a book. Hugh Fearnley-Whittingstall is one of my food heroes, care of his daring attitude to not wasting animal products, his preference for small oily fish over farmed salmon, and his nature as a fighter for the rights of chickens up and down the land (as are Jamie Oliver and Gordon Ramsey). Most of the recipes in Hugh's books can easily be adapted to suit the recommendations of *Our Natural Diet*, and many are sufficiently close to be taken outright. With other chefs, a little more thought might be required, but the key is to enjoy food and to take simple steps to make it healthier, and when something is perhaps quite problematic for health then to avoid it or at least eat it less often.

A willingness to experiment, perceptiveness and innovation are qualities that come with experience, and most recipe books can have their lists of ingredients and cooking methods adapted to maximise nutrient quality from the meals. I would rather people adapted the recipes they loved than spoil their meals by refusing outright to eat whatever they enjoyed prior to reading this book.

To summarise, this book is the next logical progression from *Human Evolution, Diet and Health*, as it assumes the groundwork has now been laid. If people are interested in the adaptations that facilitated the development of our short guts and big brains, then the information is there. This book is about a modern take on our natural health, and includes honest reviews of the latest scientific literature, regardless of whether that literature might sometimes appear contradictory; it is presented warts and all. Essentially, the notion of *'The' Natural Diet*, or anything else along such lines, is sufficient to induce some kind of spasm in the author. This book is about informed decision-making, with a few recommendations on how to adapt and refine current diets for a healthier and perhaps even 'better' way of life. It is expected to be no greater than that, and is equally hoped to be no less.

"If we wish to make a new world we have the material ready. The first one, too, was made out of chaos."

- Robert Quillen

Introduction

"The most important and urgent problems of the technology of today are no longer the satisfactions of the primary needs or of archetypal wishes, but the reparation of the evils and damages by the technology of yesterday."

- Dennis Gabor

Similar to the evils of old technologies, it can be said that common sense and accepted wisdom are the enemies of true learning and understanding. A child incessantly asking 'why' can easily beleaguer a parent, and it is perhaps a sickness of modern society that we educate children with facts and figures, teaching them how to become a better part of society – to be quiet and productive – rather than really fostering that questioning nature. Part of the problem is that, as a society, we seem to like being led, and we perceive power and authority as a sign of success. Would it not be better if, instead of trying to teach children facts, our teachers encouraged children to experiment more and find things out for themselves?

Life is too short to go through such a laborious process to answer every question, but we seem to live in a society in which it is frowned upon to ask a question, and a sign of idiocy not to know the answer. As Socrates put it "*I am the wisest man alive, for I know one thing, and that is that I know nothing*", and one of the Buddhist philosophies is that in the expert's mind the possibilities are few, whereas in the child's they are many. We seem to disassociate ourselves too readily from this childlike state, in which we have far more to learn by asking questions than by convincing ourselves we already know the answers. Life would be very dull indeed if we believed we had so little left to learn. We might as well give up reading books altogether, and dedicate our lives outside of work to watching soap operas and reality television. I would prefer a child's mind and a Meccano set any day, but maybe that is just me.

Our Natural Diet is not a book of facts scribbled out to impart knowledge. This book is far more concerned with promoting the findings of real scientists, whilst simultaneously undoing some of the damage caused by those who have dictated their pseudoscience in books and the press, and have generated a false wisdom already accepted by many. Pseudoscience refers to terms and ideas that sound 'sciencey', but which are not actually based upon real science. This could be either through the accidental misinterpretation of actual evidence, or by deliberately misleading people. In both cases there is the lack of a sound scientific rationale for providing the recommendations and ideas given. The danger is that if enough people buy into such concepts, over time there is a risk of genuine nonsense becoming the new common sense. In all cases it must surely be wrong to mislead others, particularly for the sake of personal gain and profit, but it is further damaging because it can generate a lack of trust in real science and research.

As for this book, in some cases it will be shown that the truth can be more complicated and involved than commonly thought, with research ongoing and no definitive answers yet available. In others it will be fairly clear the reality is pleasantly simple and straightforward. It would be a very sad existence to dedicate too many years to undoing some of the nonsense surrounding dietetics and nutrition, but by giving an overview of the basics and working up, we should manage to dispel the myths and introduce a better way without too much trouble.

Although not every aspect of human nutrition has been

included here, the most important areas certainly have. The message that will resonate throughout is that too much of something can be as harmful as too little, and this is even true for the foods we might imagine had no ill-effects at all. Perhaps it would be best to embark on this adventure as a whole new story, reserving judgement until the facts are in, and never being afraid to ask 'Why?'

"Our bodies are our gardens – our wills are our gardeners."
-William Shakespeare

Research, Nutrition & the Popular Press

"In all science, error precedes the truth, and it is better it should go first than last."

- Hugh Walpole

It has been said that the technology of today is here to undo the problems caused by the technology of yesterday, and it may be very much a similar issue with imparted information too. The purpose of this book is twofold. First, it is to summarise and present the latest, research-based developments in our understanding of nutrition and dietetics. Second, it is to try and undo so many of the misunderstandings and misconceptions that plague the health industry. It is no longer enough to state that carbohydrates are important, for example, but we must also now state why carbohydrates are not 'bad'.

The reason we are compelled to go through such a protracted and time-consuming step is that people with a biased and/or incomplete viewpoint have convinced others their own ideas are actually 'fact'. Hence, such misconceptions have to be clarified before we can begin to address the key issues. Traditionally, people with something to sell make their case appealing by presenting information that *seems* self-evident and yet conflicts with the accepted status quo, thus making it sexy and fashionable. This has far more to do with marketing and sales than science, evidence, health and dietary success.

Should we imagine, for example, that a recent diet bestseller, such as *The Dukan Diet*, was tested rigorously over years, with the findings compared to measures taken of equal numbers of subjects

11

with different diets, so as to demonstrate effectiveness? If such a study were conducted, who would fund the research and might that have an effect on the outcome? Let us suppose there is no high-quality, objectively critiqued, medical-journal-published research on the long-term effectiveness of *The Dukan Diet* specifically. Why would anyone follow it? If there is no adequate evidence that it works, yet the book is a bestseller, presumably enough people are willing to try it out. Why? If there is no evidence, perhaps it is because of the sales pitch – the collection of words on the front cover, back cover and in any associated press. Why believe it?

Perhaps some people assume there is sufficient evidence of a diet's effectiveness to give it a try. Maybe they did not experience the success they wanted with other diets, and simply wanted to give the next popular one a go. Possibly, what it comes down to is that some people are not really interested in the evidence for why something works, because they are content to go on trust, or at least have no reason to suppose something written or advised is not trustworthy or accurate. Even worse, maybe some people do not realise there is any alternative, and are left thinking that whatever is published in a book is the best thing they have to guide them when it comes to diet and health. One thing that should develop from this book is the realisation that the best guide for the individual is the individual himself or herself. The disturbing fact remains that a diet book can be a bestseller, followed by millions, and yet be entirely free of evidence for its effectiveness. Are there not moral and ethical issues with this – proclaiming false truths that mislead others not just into investing their money, but staking their own health and wellness on it too?

That faith and trust is a pre-requisite for 'learning' about diets and health is not right, and whilst some individuals are making an awful lot of money out of the diet industry, others are having their understanding and quite possibly their health harmed by it. There are plenty who are not even profiting from the bad advice they give, and make their recommendations under the honest belief their own knowledge is both helpful *and* accurate.   Faith, belief and a willingness for something to be true does not make it so. The sooner publishers (including individuals with websites to express their personal views) and the press accept and act upon this the better. The resources exist, but are being blocked by editors and those who think they know their market better than the market itself and those trying to do good within it. The times must change. Editors, if anything, perhaps know the market they have shaped, but it is unsettling to imagine people really prefer to be kept in the dark about their own health. There is so much information published in the academic and medical press every month, but this valuable information is not routinely reviewed and written into regular newspaper columns or magazine articles.

* * * * * * *

Part of the problem is that many people are unaware of what research really is, what hoops have to be jumped through before an investigation can begin, and what, if anything, can be interpreted from the published findings. There is insufficient scope within a book on diet to fully discuss research methods in detail, and Ben Goldacre's *Bad Science* and Edzard Ernst's *Healing, Hype or Harm?* are far more appropriate for the task. *Bad Science* addresses issues relating to how research is, and should be, conducted, how bias can render results meaningless, and how some of the more popular voices in health and nutrition have so effectively misled the public. *Healing, Hype or Harm?* is a selection of essays on complementary, alternative and integrative medicine, which describes how pseudoscience is used to misguide the public and generate a bias based upon trust and hope.

There are too many types of scientist to name, even just amongst the nutritional sciences, but broadly they could be dieticians, biologists, chemists, physiologists, urologists, toxicologists, neuroscientists, nephrologists, hepatologists, immunologists, biochemists, gerontologists, gastroenterologists, and various others. These are not necessarily scientists who set out to study nutrients and diets, but might be investigating health, a disease or some other disorder, and then examining the effects of diet or supplementation on that condition.

The term 'nutritionist' has been excluded here, because it is not a meaningful, protected term – at least not in the United Kingdom. There are no controls to stop people proclaiming themselves as nutritionists, regardless of whether they have studied nutrition at university for three years, taken a two-week course, or simply read a few magazine articles. If someone declares themselves to be a dietician, by contrast, they are expected to have a bachelor's degree in the subject at the very least, and if they have not then legal action can be taken against them. This is not the case for 'nutritionists', and so anyone who declares him or herself as such does not necessarily hold a single qualification.

So, there are scientists, such as dieticians, biochemists and physiologists, who are based within academic and research institutions, and whose job it is to perform research and publish their findings. There is not a true scientist anywhere whose job it is to have their findings published in the press. Scientific publications appear in research journals, either for a specific field of science (such as *The Journal of Lipid Science* or *The European Journal of Cancer Prevention*), a more general field (such as *The British Journal of Nutrition*), or of far broader scope (*British Medical Journal, New*

England Journal of Medicine, Nature).

Universities, university departments and individual researchers have their status improved by publishing in very good journals, and their status lowered by publishing in poor quality journals or producing no publications at all. There is typically no reward or benefit for researchers in having findings published directly into newspapers, magazines or websites. However, a university might gain popularity if it has departments producing ground-breaking research that helps the university attract students, and perhaps help in attracting organisations to fund research. Press coverage confers no academic benefit to research institutions, and most researchers should be too busy to spend their time trying to attract media attention in any case. For the member of the public wanting a greater insight into what new research is really being produced, there is a problem because the researchers are unlikely to have the time or inclination to report their findings to the press, and the press typically does not have access to the original research publications.

It might be that a department or institution likes to see some press coverage for reasons associated with public relations, but this tends to be the bane of many researchers, expected to discuss their life's work with journalists, who traditionally only want a few key statements and will then report on the work in such a way as to make it sound far more exciting, earth-shattering and juicy than it ever really was.

Science is about peering into test tubes, wasting several months investigating something that turns out to be a dead-end, or spending even more time trying to validate the reliability of measuring devices. Science is for people who have an ability to look for a problem in the smallest aspect of something, and then set about doggedly investigating this, ploughing months and years of their lives into reading and researching, applying for funding, and eventually getting some small-scale 'pilot' work underway to see if there is any scope in investigating it on a more useful and meaningful scale. Curiously, we might see this whole process as 'fun', or if not then at least highly rewarding, because we are actively doing something to improve understanding within that area of science.

So, whenever we read anything based on a scientific 'breakthrough' in the press, we should harbour some scepticism. For publication in an academic journal, the background to the original study would have been condensed down into a few paragraphs, along with a methods' section, data analysis section, a discussion of the findings and a summary or conclusion. There could have been mistakes, perhaps in the way the study was performed, especially if some of the researchers were biased, or the population they tested was very unusual and not representative of the population as a whole. In the media, whatever the original investigation was about, whatever it found (regardless of whether or not it really represents the 'truth'), was condensed down even further into a few key sentences, interpreted and edited (and probably sexed-up) by multiple journalists and editors, before finally going into the press. Simply because something was researched by proper scientists is not sufficient reason to trust that whatever ends up in the public domain is a fair reflection of that work.

A particularly relevant point raised by Ben Goldacre was that what we read in the press about health is unfairly dumbed-down. Although the offending newspapers, magazines and websites might like to claim this is because the original science is too complicated for the lay reader, this is absolutely, categorically not true, and most of us no doubt find the suggestion quite offensive. As Einstein put it, if a scientist cannot explain his or her work in clear terms, they do not really understand it themselves. It may be complicated in a book or article when it is hard to gauge the background knowledge of the readership, but this only creates a challenge and is certainly not reason to avoid attempting it in the first place.

My primary area of research is in physiology, and when it comes to areas outside of my research experience, such as geology or cosmology, for example, I have no advantage over any other 'lay' person when it comes to understanding scientific findings in those fields. But if those findings interest me, then as a human being I have the intellectual capacity to learn about those subjects. I can read some general background information, perhaps initially online or in fairly easy-going books, but then I can buy one or two more academic textbooks, and I can read some of the original research articles. I can even skip the first couple of steps and just read some free research articles in the online databases, because I will pick up enough information from those and can check anything I am unsure of on Google. There will be clear trends and debates within the research articles to inform me on which findings are reliable and which are still disputed. This whole process will not make me an expert, but it will give me an appreciable basic understanding.

Health is something important to everyone, and considering the amount of research that has been published in scientific journals over the past 150 years, the media could incorporate a fairly high standard of coverage on certain topics. But they do not. There has been no general, gradual increase in complexity on health-relevant issues, but rather just the typical, rhetorical, headline-grabbing blurb that is based more on fad and fashion than genuinely interesting research. Imagine if the economics sections of papers were like that – there would be no developing trends or depth of insight – merely headlines and the most basically worded overviews. But the economics sections are quite complex, as are the sections dealing with world affairs, fashion and sport. There are literally millions of research articles that have been published on health, and every month there are hundreds more, yet for all we see in the press there might be only one study every few months. There seems to be a gaping void between the information available to be reported on, and what is actually reported. The developing trends and complexities seem to be avoided in health as they are in no other aspect of the press.

Further, if we read a column on sports results, for example, we might be expected to know at once who team managers are, results of other recent fixtures, transfer details, and some element of the history of that team and others. Just because it would be challenging for someone with absolutely no knowledge of a particular sport or team to understand the article, this does not make it a *bad* article. Nor was the article dumbed-down for the lay reader, because, in fact, it was *assumed* the readers would be aware of the background. By contrast, almost every single article on health is dumbed-down and a 'standalone' article, because it is *assumed* that readers will not understand the background, history or related research.

The only reason the reader would not know these details is because the media itself appears disinterested, and seems to prefer publishing articles on passing fads rather than generate real awareness of important aspects of health. Of all the topics covered in the press – the world affairs, economics, fashion, health and sport – the one topic of utmost importance to the individual and their family is health, and yet that is the one area that receives the least depth and analysis.

What makes this worse, and which is another point formerly raised by Ben Goldacre, is that this state of affairs has nothing to do with available expertise in the press industry. There are plenty of individuals who have graduated from university with backgrounds in health-related fields, and who could more than adequately analyse emerging areas of interest in health and report on them. It is a travesty that the media is still driven by fads and fashion when it comes to nutrition and health, and the reader is the one left with such mixed messages and a lack of clarity. Again, *Bad Science* is a good place to start for a deeper understanding of these issues.

* * * * * * *

All the writer of any book or article can do is describe what they understand of a topic. How much of that understanding has come from rigorous hard research, and how much has come from guesswork, opinion and general craftiness might not be at all obvious. Even those who are guided purely by real scientific research are still at the mercy of their own biased interpretations, however much they might like to convince themselves and others otherwise. The inherent problem is that it is almost always second-hand information; meaning one person has become aware of something and is then passing that on to others. We have not accessed that original information ourselves, and so we put ourselves in a position where we have to *trust* the judgement of someone else.

If we were to disregard these translators and interpreters of information, and seek out the original studies ourselves, where would we begin? For anything related to diet, nutrition and health, we could do a lot worse than starting out with *PubMed*. This is an online database that indexes health and medicine-related journals. Not every article, or even every journal, is necessarily of good quality, or even accurate, but that is why an understanding of research methods is useful – to be able to separate the wheat from the chaff, as it were. Trisha Greenhalgh wrote the book *How to Read a Paper*, which describes this at a good level.

Although *PubMed* is often the first port of call for academics of health and medicine-related research, other databases include

BioMed Central, *Highwire Press*, *Web of Knowledge*, *Ovid Gateway* and even *Google Scholar*. It would be worth finding *PubMed* on a search engine, and then going through the tutorials available on the homepage. Try searching for something of interest, such as free radicals, oxidative stress, a particular supplement, or a particular food.

The first thing to bear in mind when reading a paper is that it was written by a human being who wanted to get his or her paper published. There might have been mistakes in their methods. They might have found very little effect of their treatment or intervention, but they might go on to make any effect seem greater than it really was. They might have made mistakes in their testing procedures, which they realised and omitted from the write-up. The real strength of a scientific article, however, is in the 'peer-review'. This is the process whereby researchers submit their article for publication and it is first distributed amongst a group of experienced researchers (peers) in that field. Their individual reviews should highlight any bias, miscalculations, errors in measurements or methodological oversights, and return the article to the authors for corrections. Alternatively, the journal editors may simply decide the piece is not appropriate for publication in their journal at all. Hence, there is some credibility to a paper published in a good journal.

In the discussion section of a research article, the authors have to put their findings in the context of what other researchers have found. In doing so they will be limited by the effectiveness of their own literature searches, and may have missed out important studies which conflicted with their own findings (they might even have deliberately ignored them). Also, if a paper was published last year, the literature search would have been limited to everything published up to a few months before. What about studies published more recently? What about studies currently underway, or those that are being developed at the moment?

There is never enough information in a single paper to grant the reader a full and complete perspective of that area of science, as it stands today. The best we can do is to read a number of research papers, and try and develop an understanding of what has led to emerging trends. For many of us that will simply not fit into the time we have available, but if we read something important in the press, we can at least conclude that the reality is probably far more complex than is being made out, and we could – if we wanted to – go a little further in trying to better understand the topic. Perhaps it might interest readers to know the manuscript of this book was passed over to peers for recommendations, and so in a similar way this book should be stronger because of that process. Unfortunately there is no requirement for this approach, and no team of researchers available to all publishers to provide such a service.

The validity of a claim – whether in a book, research paper or newspaper article – might be particularly important if we are thinking of reacting in some way. For example, a few recent investigations have supported the use of ketogenic diets for treating certain types of cancer. Before a cancer-sufferer could act on that, he or she would need to know whether the type of cancer they have could be affected positively or negatively by making such a drastic change to their diet. That would involve reading more studies and seeking advice from the relevant medical specialists.

On a less dramatic level, perhaps a newspaper article touted a particular supplement as being the new best thing for improving libido, and that was something that just happened to appeal. We might want to know if the finding reported was accurate, or if money would be wasted for nothing. Perhaps, if taken for a prolonged period, the supplement might actually have deleterious effects on the health of blood vessels, increasing the risk of male impotence, or reducing the likelihood of reaching climax. How many studies had been conducted and over what period of time? If the supplement has only been studied for a two-week period, then nobody knows what the long-term effects might be if taken for a month, three months or a year. How do we decide if something is both safe and effective?

It might be interesting to note that studies of supplements are more likely to demonstrate the supplement worked if the manufacturing company funded the investigation. In fact, it is very difficult to find published research on supplements that has not been funded by the manufacturers.

New supplements come onto the market almost monthly, so why would a researcher want to dedicate his or her working life to investigating a supplement, when a long-term study is rendered worthless because a new pill will come onto the market and replace it? How do you generate a living for yourself as a researcher in this field, unless you happen to find funding, and presumably the only people interested in funding such research are the supplement companies themselves? Fortunately, researchers are expected to declare within their publications if their studies were funded and if so by whom, and it would be very poor practice not to admit to these, as the publication could later be withdrawn if any such inconsistencies were exposed.

* * * * * * *

Authors of diet books, including this one, should be assumed to be biased, using research only to support their own preconceived ideas. This is particularly obvious when a step is missing between the actual research produced and the message given. As an example, there is a book that recommends people adjust their diets according to their blood type. There are literally hundreds of different blood groups, and the common types most people are familiar with (ABO and rhesus) are the best known because the consequences of receiving a transfusion from the wrong type can be disastrous. Nevertheless, there are hundreds of different blood groups in all, and we simply tend to know less about the others because the effects are not so serious if we receive a transfusion of a type different to our own.

A blood type refers to the immune factors on the red blood cells, which is determined by genetic and other factors. So, it is not at all difficult to find hundreds of research papers that have investigated different blood types in regard to immune function. Similarly, there are many hundreds of research papers on the interactions between diet and the immune system. However, to make the leap from diet to blood type to health and weight loss is ridiculous, and not supported at all. In the back of the book in question there are hundreds of research articles referenced, mostly on either diet and health or blood type and health, but when the titles are read it is clear there is no good evidence for a link between diet and blood type, or at least not in a sense that the book is proclaiming. It appears at first glance to be supported by a wealth of evidence, but actually it is nothing more than pseudoscience.

Really, if we were given a hundred journal articles about a particular aspect of nutrition, then we should all come up with the same basic summary and conclusions. The writer is only another interpreter, and his or her role is important because life is sometimes too short for everyone to be expected to read up everything on a subject. But when a writer decides not to give a fair appraisal of the literature, and instead wants to manipulate the available research to suit his or her own needs, creating conclusions and recommendations that are not backed-up by the total evidence, then there is a serious moral and ethical issue. That this is done to create a new, fashionable approach, either to sell a book or sell some supplements is deeply unsettling.

Decisions should be based upon evidence, and if all readers of this book were to read the references then they ought to arrive at similar conclusions. One problem is that bias creeps in; so even what we read tends to be tainted by what we think we already know. A good scientist is someone who supposes to know nothing but the scientific method. Understanding how to research is far more valuable than knowing what has already been researched. Because of this, hypotheses are very, very precious, and often easily disproved.

It is worth noting that nothing can ever be *proven* by science, only *disproved*. Simply because the Sun rises each day in the east, this does not mean it will tomorrow, because there could be some irregular celestial phenomenon of which we have been hitherto unaware. As soon as a scientist decides to believe something, they are setting themselves up to be disproved. A hypothesis or theory can only ever be *supported* by evidence, but it takes only one exception to disprove it.

Sometimes the hypothesis has to be refined according to new information, and sometimes it has to be disregarded altogether and a new hypothesis formulated. Therein lies the beauty of science. Every day we can learn something new, and we can embrace that and enjoy it because we are not chained to old beliefs. We want progress rather than tradition, and that progress comes from a consistency in more and more evidence supporting a particular theory, with refinements creeping in whenever new evidence is found. It is hoped that each of the chapters in this book can be improved from one edition to the next, as new research develops and improves upon the original. Again, due to the wealth of supporting evidence it is most likely that progress will be in the form of subtle refinements, rather than the total abandonment of the original.

There is now so much evidence for the simple and straightforward approach included here that it is unlikely any of the general recommendations will be overturned, but it is important that any changes are embraced and encouraged as part of the nature of science. In this regard the pseudoscientists are easy to spot, because they will use the research to *prove* their arguments, whereas a scientist would rather *disprove* their ideas so as to develop a better, stronger, and more accurate understanding.

What the real research tends to demonstrate is that no foods need be absolutely avoided. Evidence also shows that our diets, in general, have taken a turn for the worse over recent decades, and there is plenty of scope for improvement. Perhaps the most important approach, therefore, is to determine – based upon the evidence – those dietary factors we can adapt, abandon or improve. In any case, a positive desire to make changes for the benefit of health is vital, and such an aspiration requires direction derived from salient, unpolluted, and accurate details about health and nutrition. As Carl Sagan put it, "*Science is a way of thinking much more than it is a body of knowledge*". Thus, we ought to be prepared to fine-tune our approach to health as more information comes to light, but it is hoped the research included in this book is general enough to remain accurate for some considerable time to come.

Our Natural Diet

"Health is a state of complete physical, mental and social
well-being, and not merely the absence of disease or infirmity."
- World Health Organisation

For Health

A key principle of this book is that health is the foundation for everything. If a diet lacks quality then eventually cravings will reign supreme and cause problems. Either the cravings cause the person to revert back to a less healthy existence, or else the person doggedly suffers their cravings and their quality of life is harmed as a result. Health is as much about the mind as the body, and shortcomings in the health of one will eventually affect the other. Having a good diet is about ensuring the body is supported by good nutrition, and that there are few, if any, compromises as far as our health is concerned.

Although this book is naturally focussed on diet, it should be absolutely clear that overall good health requires sufficient physical activity, and a limitation of negative psychological stressors. Health is also affected by environmental and genetic factors, and an awareness of these can be of some use. Some people will expose themselves to chemical hazards whether they work in polluted cities, in industrial manufacturing plants, or even on modern farms. These are the compromises we make in order to provide homes, food and security, but the penalty can be respiratory disorders and worse. Fortunately, improved measuring techniques and increased awareness of environmental pollutants is helping reduce the magnitude of these problems.

It is a particularly wretched aspect of human nature that if someone we know has a negative experience; some individuals will use this as their excuse to denounce all aspects of health and medicine. Part of the problem lies in our nature to project the experiences of others onto ourselves. In research we would argue that 'data is not the plural of anecdote'. One person, as an individual, is an inordinately complex organism, and whatever befalls one, or a hundred, or even a billion, might not happen to us personally.

We have probably all seen a cold or flu be passed amongst colleagues, family members or friends, but not have it affect us, only to succumb the next time one goes around. We cannot make perfect predictions or guarantees, but we can do everything to tip the balance of health in our favour. Some people contract fewer colds than others, or are affected by them for less time. Some people recover from heart disease, and some people contract cancers which are effectively treated, allowing them to pursue a full and rich life. In the grand scheme of things, if life can be better for being healthy, with us feeling more full of life, more energetic, less lethargic, and less susceptible to illness, then we probably owe it to ourselves to pursue this. If food tastes good and life feels better for the process, then there cannot conceivably be a downside.

The growing popularity of diet and health books, health and fitness magazines, health products and health and fitness clubs, demonstrates we are interested in this. Many of us like the idea that we can obtain some higher level of living, in which health is more than just the absence of disease, but rather is a condition of being in which we can thrive and really feel better in ourselves. There is a magnificent difference between simply being free from illness and actually thriving. If we eat the right foods, enjoy a physically active lifestyle, reduce our daily stresses, sleep just enough and surround ourselves with a healthy environment, we should be able to enjoy life to the full. There are no magic pills or potions, no real superfoods and no short-cuts to any aspect of health. But that is not to say achieving full health is anything but straightforward, enjoyable and easily achieved.

For Looks

◆ No animal in the wild would be alive if it had not been born with a system of internal cues to aid survival. There is no lion that chooses to eat meat because he thinks he ought to do so, and no wildebeest consuming grass simply because all the other wildebeest are doing so.

Our continuing survival is the result of homeostatic mechanisms that respond to change. If we feel hungry, we eat, if we feel thirsty we drink, and if we need salt then we desire salty foods (we also excrete dilute urine, so that the overall balance of water to salt improves). Perhaps people like to be told what to eat and how much to drink because we do not realise how much better it is to be guided by our instincts. But then, our experiences and what we have available also influence our desires for food. So many modern foods, including processed meats or grains, are high in energy but low in nutritional value, meaning we overeat but can remain under-nourished, making us want to eat more. If we seek out more of these nutrient-poor foods, then we end up with a lot of energy going in that is stored as fat, but lacking in the nutrients required to support our immune systems, promote a healthy appearance, and help us to feel energetic rather than lethargic.

If someone wishes to lose weight, it is fairly easy to shed any excess on a more natural diet, and very difficult to gain fat, simply because the foods are very high in nutritive value. On the other hand, if someone wants to increase their muscle mass or tone-up, that is just a matter of performing the right amount, type and intensity of resistance training, whilst ensuring the diet delivers sufficient proteins and enough energy. All such things are easily managed. What is more, there is some evidence to support the idea that the sorts of foods recommended in this book are the sorts of foods most beneficial for promoting healthy skin, hair and nails, too.

For Life

It is intended that any changes this approach to diet promotes will facilitate real, noticeable benefits. Broadly, the foods recommended here are fresh fruits, fresh vegetables, fresh meat and fresh fish. Some foods are delicately recommended against, and where these were initially staples of the diet it is essential their substitution is a gradual process. Some people might find it perfectly straightforward to overhaul their diet, if this seems necessary, whereas others might find that meal choices become limited. This should not be the case, as the sorts of foods recommended are full of flavour, but if preparing them and eating so much of them is a novelty, then it is better to do this gradually rather than all in one go. One should not be preparing the same food every night of the week, and nor should one have to consult a recipe book for every meal. The happy medium might come from sticking with some of the foods that are less than ideal, whilst gradually experimenting and introducing the healthier alternatives, prepared in different styles and including some new foods.

There are no styles of cooking that need be avoided, but

generally an increase in healthier cooking methods and a reduction of less healthy ones would be reasonable. For example, Italian meals based on fish or chicken, particularly with a tomato-based sauce, are far healthier, more flavoursome, and richer in nutrients than the more basic breads, pastas and pizzas, but there is no reason to totally rule anything out. A similar approach will work for all other world cuisines, so from the outset it is important to appreciate that the recommendations are towards innovation and experimentation, rather than outright restriction or avoidance.

As already discussed, it would be ridiculous to have a recipe book to accompany this one, as it would suggest confinement into however many recipes could be thought up. Really, almost any meal can be made healthier, and understanding the recommendations within this book will help ensure any recipe in any recipe book is as healthy as can be. When this is not realistic, because the recipe really does have so few redeeming foods, then eating it less often seems the most reasonable approach.

Carbohydrates

"If more of us valued food and cheer and song above hoarded gold,
it would be a merrier world."

- J. R. R. Tolkien

Carbohydrate is a collective term for sugars, starches and dietary fibres, and any plant food will contain a variety of these. The composition of a fruit or vegetable will differ according to type, ripeness, soil quality and various other factors. A sugar is a fairly simple carbohydrate molecule, whereas a starch is made up of a combination of these. Carbohydrates can also be described as simple or complex (really the same idea as sugars and starches), and refined or unrefined (according to the level of processing).

The digestive processes break carbohydrates down into simpler forms, such as glucose – a key energy source for our cells. Carbohydrate foods are typically sources of dietary fibres, which are important for gut health and provide us with energy, as well as providing our gut bacteria with energy too. The type and amount of fibre will vary between carbohydrate sources. Plant foods, particularly fruits and vegetables rather than cereal grains[*], are also sources of vitamins, minerals and other important nutrients.

Dietary carbohydrates mostly come from plant-source foods, with the notable exception of the sugars in dairy products. All types of fruits, vegetables and cereal grains contain carbohydrates. Aside from the sugars within fruits, the only sugar we would have experienced during most of our evolutionary history would have been honey, and

---

[*] i.e., wheat, oats, barley, rye

31

that would have been only seasonally available. Due to our modern tastes, many common fruits have been carefully selected for their sweetness, meaning they have a higher sugar content, are lower in fibre, and generally have fewer seeds than wild varieties.

Modern convenience has led to the increased popularity of grain foods, due to their ease of preparation and low cost. Breakfast cereals are poured from a packet, sandwiches are made from pre-sliced bread, and pasta is tipped into boiling water. Vegetables, by contrast, need to be washed and chopped before they can be cooked, which, combined with their cost and limited shelf life, has meant cereal grains have replaced them as the main source of carbohydrates for many, with dairy foods coming second. Other carbohydrates included in the diet might be sweets, chocolate, biscuits and cakes, which are made from a combination of cereal grains, refined sugar and fats.

That cereals, pasta and even bread outlast vegetables is a sign these are not biologically active substances. Vegetables are rich sources of important bacteria (prebiotics), dietary fibres, starchy carbohydrates and a plethora of essential nutrients. Cereal grains are a peculiar food, because they have to be so heavily processed by comparison to vegetables, after which they tend to be so bereft of useful nutrients it is common for breakfast cereals to have a few token vitamins and minerals added to them. Because breads, pastas and cereals are so limited in nutrients, they are limited in flavour too, which is why they are usually combined with other foods.

From an evolutionary perspective, our short guts, resident bacteria and the types of enzymes we have are simply inefficient at breaking cereal grains down, as is the case with other primates. Small birds, insects and weevils like cereal grains, and indeed can thrive on them, but large mammals cannot. We can live on them, provided we have other sources of essential nutrients, but otherwise their benefits (outside of general convenience) are limited.

It is quite likely that many modern diseases have been generated by our substitution of fruits and vegetables with nutrient- and digestion-poor cereal grain foods. The plant nutrients within fruits and vegetables come in thousands of varieties. These *phytochemicals* are important for protecting our hearts and blood vessels, and for defending us against potentially harmful substances in the blood and cells. They are also protective against some cancers, various disorders, and age-related degenerative conditions. Although cereal grain foods supply basic carbohydrates, they do not have the additional benefit of those phytonutrients, and including them at the expense of fruits and vegetables is far from ideal.

This is not, however, to assert that cereal grains should be avoided entirely. The most important point is that vegetable intake should not be compromised by the convenience of cereal grain foods. Rather than breakfast cereals, breads and pastas being the staples, with vegetables relegated to a mere garnish at best, it would be beneficial to try and correct this.

Another means of increasing our intake of nutrient-rich carbohydrates is when snacking. Snack foods based on cereal grains – such as pastries, biscuits and cakes – could easily be replaced with a variety of different fruits. Fruits are filled with protective and health-promoting nutrients, whereas pastries, cakes and biscuits are sufficient to keep us alive, but aside from that contain few (if any) useful nutrients and have a far greater potential to do harm. To avoid a fluffy ending to that point, the high concentration of sugars in typical snack foods can promote obesity and diabetes, whilst content of certain vegetable oils might promote cancer development, negatively affect the healing process, and negatively impact on the cardiovascular system. Fruit, by contrast, helps protect against diabetes and some cancers, promotes efficient healing and supports the health of the heart and blood vessels.

The goal need not be to avoid sugary snack foods entirely, but rather to ensure they contribute only a minor proportion to the overall diet. The nutrients in fruits and vegetables are protective against the negatives associated with grain foods, so it seems that by eating more fruits and vegetables, so we can enjoy a few more of the treats whilst reducing any risk of ill-health. Conversely, a diet where breads, pasta, cereals, biscuits and cakes are consumed most days a week would best be corrected, both because of the problems these can cause to the gut, cardiovascular system and overall health, and because of all the nutrients being missed through the limiting of fruit and vegetable intake.

One elephant, formerly peering nonchalantly about in the corner of the room, and which has subsequently loomed more closely to the forefront, is the mammoth subject of dairy foods. In our modern diets, the majority of carbohydrate comes from cereal grains, with dairy foods often being the second highest carbohydrate-contributor. Fruits and vegetables combined make up a very poor twenty-ish percent, despite their being the only source of carbohydrates of our Palaeolithic ancestors.

Dairy foods, like cereal grains, are not a part of our evolutionary, physiological heritage. No Palaeolithic humans would have consumed milk after weaning, and the inclusion of milk as we have it now is really a cultural adaptation. We might choose to dislike it as a carbohydrate because it is an unusual sugar for adults, but in fact the topic is so elephantine that it deserves its own chapter, particularly as it naturally leads on to the subject of bone health[*].

Researchers of Palaeolithic nutrition have reported that the carbohydrate intake of our Stone-age ancestors would have been approximately 35% (although this figure would have fluctuated

---

[*] Hence there are separate chapters on Human Milk, Dairy and Bone Health

widely according to location and time of year)[1,2]. If we were to substitute our cereal grain foods for fruits and vegetables, and exclude all added sugars and dairy foods, then our modern carbohydrate intake would naturally be reduced to about this amount, and with no greater level of thought being required[1,2].

* * * * * * *

When we eat a natural source of carbohydrates, such as a fruit or vegetable, that item is a neat package of different carbohydrates, thousands of different types of plant chemicals, plus water. Many of those phytochemicals have been found to have important effects on the human body, including prevention of – and protection against – various diseases, illnesses and disorders. They help protect our blood and our cells, take care of our vision and other senses, and just generally do good deeds to support health throughout the body. The water content is a valuable addition to our daily fluid intake, and helps ensure we remain adequately hydrated. The carbohydrate content provides energy to support our cells in their activities, whether they be involved in muscular contraction or fuelling our active minds.

Digestion of carbohydrate begins in the mouth and continues along the length of the digestive tract, including the stomach and along the intestine. Some fibres cannot be easily broken down by the actions of our own enzymes, but our guts contain a variety of useful bacteria that do. Some fibres are not broken down at all, and instead act as a sponge as they travel along the intestine, cleaning up our interiors as they pass, but unfortunately gathering up useful nutrients too. Digestion is highly adapted process, but not a perfect one.

Once carbohydrates enter the blood the next step is to have

that carbohydrate driven into cells, either for use or storage. The usable form of carbohydrate is glucose, and much of the digestive process is involved in breaking carbohydrate down into this form. So, we consume some carbohydrates and our blood glucose levels rise. Cells within our pancreas are then stimulated to release insulin, which is essential for transporting glucose into most cells (there are some exceptions). All cells within the body can use glucose, and it is particularly important for the brain[*] and is used as a fuel during activity. There are alternatives, but glucose is the fuel of choice. Mammals use glucose to fuel their brains and their muscles, and in terms of our natural diets, this is what we have predominantly experienced.

So our blood glucose levels rise and then insulin drives that glucose into cells, causing levels to drop. In fact, because the body reacts in an imprecise manner, blood glucose levels tend to drop below their normal, resting values. This is partly responsible for the post-meal fatigue that can affect us. When our blood glucose levels are low we feel deprived of energy, and by feeling lethargic we behave less energetically, and this helps us to preserve the little glucose we have available in the blood. So, we stop releasing insulin because the blood glucose levels are now too low, and another hormone, glucagon, is released from the pancreas instead. Glucagon is involved in increasing blood glucose levels, mainly by releasing what is stored in the liver. Following subsequent, ever-smaller fluctuations above and below resting levels, blood glucose levels become balanced again. How much of each hormone is released and over how long will depend upon the amount of glucose in the blood, which itself will depend upon meal composition and amount, and efficiency of cells to receive glucose.

---

[*] Perhaps interestingly, the cells of the brain do not require insulin to transport glucose into them, making them an exception

Refined sugars have already been partially broken down through processing, so they do not need our bodies to do very much more with them, and they enter the blood rapidly. As a result there is a high concentration of glucose in the blood soon after consuming a meal containing refined sugars. This leads to a high insulin response, in turn causing glucose to disappear rapidly from the blood, eliciting a far more noticeable level of fatigue than when carbohydrates are released more slowly (as would occur following ingestion of unrefined carbohydrates). So, fruits and vegetables move into the blood more slowly than most breakfast cereals, cakes, biscuits, chocolate and sweets. It is unlikely this is news to anyone, but at least this is the process explained.

A diet too high in refined carbohydrates increases the risk of insulin resistance and diabetes. Insulin resistance refers to an inefficiency of insulin to drive glucose into storage locations, meaning more insulin is required to do this than in someone healthy. Long-term, this resistance can develop and worsen to become type 2 diabetes, in which the pancreas is unable to release sufficient insulin to effectively restore glucose levels following a meal. The reason it is associated with refined carbohydrates in particular is that these cause such markedly increased blood glucose concentrations. The carbohydrates in unrefined foods, particularly vegetables, are typically good sources of different fibres, which slow digestion and absorption, meaning glucose enters the blood more gradually and less insulin is required to maintain balance.

The opposite of insulin resistance is insulin sensitivity, which refers to the body's ability to use only a small amount of insulin to maintain normal blood glucose levels. Being overweight is associated with insulin resistance, whereas being lean and muscular is associated with insulin sensitivity. Exercising with weights has been shown to improve insulin sensitivity, thereby decreasing insulin resistance and helping to protect against diabetes.

The speed at which glucose levels rise following a meal can be estimated according to the food's glycaemic index (G.I.) or glycaemic load (G.L.), or at least that was the idea. The glycaemic index came about in 1981, as a means to measure the effect of a carbohydrate food on blood glucose levels, by comparing 100 grams of that food with 100 grams of a reference food (such as glucose or white bread). The idea of glycaemic load was developed in 1997, and was intended to be a more useful tool, because it adjusted the G.I. value according to realistic serving sizes, rather than the standard 100 grams. Because of this, and research demonstrating G.I. alone is not effective for predicting the true effect of a carbohydrate meal on glucose levels, the glycaemic load became favoured.

However, calculating glycaemic load is still an imperfect tool, because it is dependant upon the consumption of carbohydrate-based foods only, and suffers inaccuracies due to individual variability and the effects of consuming carbohydrates with other foods. Further, the serving sizes may not reflect actual consumption. Ice cream, for example, appears to have quite a low G.L., and yet if people consume a quantity greater than that of the actual serving size included in the tests, the effect on blood glucose levels will be different. So, although glycaemic load is an improvement to the glycaemic index, it still suffers from the assumptions that are useful for research purposes, but are less transferable to the needs of the individual.

Further, the concentration of glucose in the blood is not the only detail of relevance. Dairy foods, including milk, yoghurt and ice cream, all have a far more pronounced effect on insulin levels than would be expected based upon glycaemic load alone. This means the short-term effects of these foods would probably be a greater feeling of fatigue and tiredness, compared with the same amount of other carbohydrates with a supposedly similar G.L. Long-term, the consequences could include an increased risk of insulin resistance and ultimately diabetes, and in fact fructose – another sugar effective at raising insulin above expected levels[*] – is used to induce insulin resistance in laboratory rodents.

It seems that both G.I. and G.L. were tools developed as a scientific exercise only, with limited transferability to the real world. As with many apparently scientific tools advocated to dieters and others interested in nutrition and health, their worth is extremely limited. Really, it is just a complicated way of showing that different carbohydrates have different effects on the blood. The value of such a list, however, becomes severely limited as soon as different types of carbohydrates are consumed with other carbohydrates, proteins, fats and fluids. The simplest guide is to recommend eating meals that seem reasonable in quantity and composition. If we feel hungry after eating, then we should eat more, whereas if we feel full then we should probably have eaten less. If we feel particularly tired after a meal, then we ought to reduce the total carbohydrate content next time, and if that leaves us feeling hungry then we should compensate by eating more proteins and fats.

This should be a perfectly sensible and logical approach. The problem is that elements of science, whether misinterpreted or misunderstood, have been so commonly recommended by people who do not fully understand the real use of the research, that we might feel uneasy as if something is very wrong with turning our backs to the tables, charts, lists and equations. Well, and here is the rub: all those tables, charts, lists and equations were developed to give researchers an improved understanding of the *average* effect of a type of food on

---

[*] In addition to G.I. and G.L., we also have the Insulinaemic Index, which is a measure of the amount of insulin released for a given amount of a particular food. Dairy foods and fructose produce an insulin response proportionately much higher than their blood glucose response

the body. That is, the effect of a fairly average example of an average food, taken in an average quantity, on its own rather than with other foods, on the average person. They are not testing the actual food items, in the real quantities, prepared in exactly the same way as what we – as individuals and not as an average – are consuming in a particular meal, at a particular time of a particular day. No matter how refined, detailed and impressive the scientific tools become, unless we have someone actually taking blood samples from us minute-by-minute following every meal, science will *never ever* be as perceptive, intelligent, understanding or exceptional as we are at knowing the effects of the foods we eat on our blood glucose levels.

If we really wanted to, we could measure our glucose levels, but all we need to know is that if we feel unusually tired after a carbohydrate-rich meal, then we have probably overdone it, whereas if we feel hungry we probably ought to have eaten a little more. The brain is a highly complex organ, adapted over millions of years to ensure the body remains within healthy limits, and when these limits are approached or exceeded, some internal cue will let us know to eat more, to eat less next time, or to eat differently. This is far more complex than any blood test, and certainly more relevant to us than any table, chart or graph we could ever be (mis-)guided by.

If we decide to change our normal daily habits, we will be able to do the fine-tuning far better by being aware of how our body responds to those meals, than by attempting to count calories or measure glycaemic load. Do we feel more tired or more energetic than usual? Are we still hungry half an hour later? The research is there to support general choices, such as through the recommendations to reduce intake of refined sugars, cereal grains and dairy foods, and to replace those foods with fruits and vegetables. The research can also be used to guide preference of farming method (organic or not), packaging (plastics, jars, no packaging), preservation (pickling, dried, fresh), processing (no processing, concentrate-derived), and preparation method (raw, cooked). That is all profoundly useful information, but to try and take that further, to the point of calculating calorie requirements, precise effects of foods on the blood, and anything else along similar lines, will actually be imprecise in the case of any individual who is not the impossible average.

Dietary Fibres

"*Effective health care depends on self-care; this fact is currently heralded as if it were a discovery.*"

-Ivan Illich

Dietary fibre is non-starchy plant material, which is mostly resistant to digestion from our own enzymes along the digestive tract. Instead, fibres can be broken down by the bacteria within our guts, and the extent to which this happens will depend on the species of plant, how the food was prepared (including processing and cooking times and methods), what else comprised the meal, and individual differences[3]. This is so much the case that comparisons and predictions based solely on fibre type and structural properties are likely to be over-simplistic[3] and inaccurate as a result. Fibres can pass along the gut and act as a sponge, holding onto water and acting as a structural frame upon which bacteria can act[4].

The effect of different fibres is still a matter for investigation, although it is currently understood there are three main categories: soluble fibre, insoluble fibre, and swollen, sponge-like fibres[10]. Fibres reduce the rate – and sometimes the extent – of absorption of some nutrients. This can reduce the total bioaccessibility[*] of nutrients, because either the plant nutrients themselves are bound onto these fibres, or else fats are held on the fibres and unavailable for the nutrients to bind onto for transport across the gut[10], as is required in the case of fat-soluble vitamins.

Dietary fibres are an interesting area of current research,

---

[*] There is a separate chapter on bioaccessibility and bioavailability

because we are still attempting to fully understand the different types of fibre and their fates within the body. Research is also comparing the different types of fibres in wheat, oats and vegetables. Historically, the advice has been that wheat is the preferable source, but a few fairly alarming case studies and a greater breadth of research has begun to question earlier assumptions[5].

Non-starch vegetables, which are all vegetables except grains, potatoes and roots, appear to be the most beneficial, in that they perform the greatest number of useful actions within the body. Further, fruits and vegetables contain far more fibre than cereal grains, despite fibre-poor, refined grains contributing the vast majority of carbohydrates in our modern, westernised diets.

* * * * * * *

Flowering plants can be divided into two main groups: monocot and dicot. The distinctions between the two groups are somewhat fuzzy, but general differences relate to the structure of the embryos, the directions of veins in the leaves, and different features of the pollen and the flowers themselves. As mentioned in *Human Evolution, Diet and Health*, the group of primates that includes the monkeys, apes and ourselves is very good at digesting the dicot plant foods, and very poor at digesting many of the monocot plants. Our ability to digest a particular food is governed by the products we have to break the food down, such as enzymes, stomach acid, and gut bacteria. Our guts became very short because our diet featured high-quality foods that required only limited processing. The majority of monocot plants were not readily available to us in Africa, Asia or Europe during our evolutionary pasts, and so the ability to digest those foods would have been as useful to us then as the ability to digest moon dust.

Although not the only monocot plants in our modern diets, rice, rye, corn, barley, maize, millet, oats and wheat are the most prevalent sources of carbohydrate for most people, and they are the ones we cannot effectively break down. Fortunately, our evolutionary pasts did give us access to a few monocot plants, such as bananas, and others are consumed in such small quantities, already heavily processed by chopping, crushing and cooking, that they are less of an issue for digestion, such as garlic, onions and ginger.

As we are finding with far too many aspects of modern living (in particular those relating to diet and lifestyle), the convenience does not always give us the best of all possible worlds. As a species we tend to favour sweet foods, and foods with particular flavours and appearances. We do not like too much pulp, seeds or pips in our fruits and vegetables, and as a result these have been selectively farmed for generations to ensure they match consumer expectations. Something, naturally, had to give, and total fibre content was one such thing.

The fruits and vegetables commercially available today contain, on average, less than a third of the total fibre content of the wild varieties consumed by modern hunter-gatherer groups. Even worse, our cultivated vegetables (along with cereal grains) contain phytic acid, which inhibits the absorption of minerals. Phytic acid is broken down during the cooking process, and this is a good reason not to have a diet based largely upon the consumption of raw vegetables. Fruit is fine, as fruits are not significant sources of phytic acid, and perhaps some raw vegetables each day would do more good than harm, but overall raw vegetables should not be considered favourable to cooked.

Wild vegetables do not contain such high levels of this acid. Our modern tastes have facilitated a decreased fibre content within vegetables, and the phytic acid has reduced the availability of minerals, especially when compared with wild, uncultivated varieties. It should be pointed out that many of the phytochemicals in vegetables can be absorbed without the necessity for cooking, with minerals being a particular exception, and there are some benefits of consuming raw vegetables, but in any case all nutrients are better absorbed with more processing (chopping, crushing, blending, etc.). The phytic acid content interferes with mineral absorption in particular.

Although research into the different types of fibre and their effects is still in its infancy, useful findings have been made. Fibre types are difficult to categorise because of their different effects. A fairly old (1991) study[6] reported that an increase in soluble fibre (oat bran) led to a decrease in total and LDL cholesterol in men with high cholesterol levels, whereas levels were unchanged in men who increased their intake of wheat bran.

The fibre content of fruits and vegetables is higher than that of cereal grains, although it seems the importance of fibres from fruits and vegetables has been slow to reach medical advisers (although the evidence is easily accessible). Individuals with gut disorders can still be given the generic recommendation to increase intake of any fibre, including from wheat-based sources. One large-scale study published in the *Lancet*[7], found that wheat fibre antagonised irritable bowel syndrome (IBS) in sufferers, and a review paper[5] concluded that the automatic recommendation to increase fibre intake in those suffering with IBS needed to be challenged. That these papers were published around fifteen years ago, and wheat fibre is still recommended to people with IBS suggests people are either reluctant to change their ways or simply resistant to learning.

Fibre is beneficial, but the type of fibre is important as all do not have equal effects, and the fibres from fruits and vegetables are far more beneficial than those from cereal grains. The intake of fibres from fruits, vegetables and oats has been associated with decreased total and LDL cholesterol levels[1,6,8]. An insufficient intake of fibre has been associated with the initiation or exacerbation of constipation, appendicitis, haemorrhoids, deep vein thrombosis, varicose veins, diverticulitis, hiatal hernia and gastrointestinal reflux[1].

* * * * * * *

Fibre interacts with other nutrients in the diet, affecting the overall absorption of both macronutrients and micronutrients. As fibre content increases, fat and protein digestibility decreases[9], but so far this has been poorly researched, with fibres coming from multiple sources, and little understanding developed regarding the interactions amongst different fibre types with different fats. Two important findings of this research have been that there are significant differences between individuals consuming identical meals, and the difficult to predict effects of fibre on total metabolisable energy mean that estimates of calorie intake from a meal become very imprecise[9].

Really, the generic use of the term dietary fibre needs to be questioned, because this is over-simplistic and non-specific. The different fibres in fruits and vegetables, for example, exhibit a diverse range of effects on the body, and because so many foods contain fibres it is unhelpful to imply the benefits occur from all types. Fruits and vegetables confer all the benefits of fibres from cereal grains, but have additional positive effects on gut health and blood cholesterol levels[4].

The benefits from plant foods include improved cardiovascular and gastrointestinal health, maintained health of organs and other tissues, and protection against cancers, age-related degenerative conditions, and diabetes. Further, plant foods offer the healthiest source of carbohydrate for energy.

That we cannot utilise all of what we eat, and that some components inhibit the absorption of others, is because these are natural products we choose to eat, rather than foodstuffs *designed* to work perfectly with such a complex organism as a mammalian body. All this really means is that we need to consume more rather than fewer fruits and vegetables, in as great a variety as is available, with benefits to consuming some raw, some cooked and some pureed. Any one strategy in isolation is never going to be as beneficial as including in the diet a variety of plant foods, prepared using a variety of methods.

* * * * * * *

Although our cultivated plant foods might not be as high in fibre as their wild counterparts, it is important we ensure we eat plenty of the fruits and vegetables available to us, because this will provide far more useful and valuable fibres than those found in other carbohydrate foods. By exchanging cereal grains with fruits and vegetables, we will be making a profoundly positive step towards better health and reducing our risks of developing disease.

Most importantly, the reduction in intake of some foods, and substitutions of others, is a matter requiring a gradual approach, consisting of trial and error and a willingness to experiment with new foods and recipes. In particular, it is likely that more success will be gained from altering one meal and one snack at a time, especially as preparing vegetables takes a little longer and can require a little more thought than preparing cereal grain foods. It is something worth getting right, and ensuring it is an approach we want to stick with.

These and related concepts will be discussed further and expanded upon elsewhere in the book, due to the crossovers between different food groups and other dietary factors.

Fruits & Vegetables

"A table, a chair, a bowl of fruit and a violin;
what else does a man need to be happy?"
- Albert Einstein

In modern diets, nutrient- and fibre-poor refined sugars, nutrient-poor and poorly digested cereal grains, and dairy foods have mostly replaced nutrient- and fibre-rich fruits and vegetables. This change has been associated with increased risk of some cancers, increased risk of insulin resistance and diabetes, reduced defences against cellular damage, reduced healing and increased risk of damage to the heart and blood vessels. Furthermore, our modern tastes have led to fruits and vegetables that have been selected to have lower fibre content than their uncultivated relatives. Correcting the imbalances requires a gradual but determined approach to reducing intake of refined sugars and dairy products, and substituting cereal grain foods with fruits and vegetables.

Fruit and vegetable intake is associated with reduced risks of cardiovascular disease, some diseases of the eye, certain degenerative diseases[11], and various cancers[12,13]. That fruits and vegetables are beneficial is unlikely to be news to anyone, although the underlying mechanisms, the importance of variety and the relevance of different cooking methods might be. Something of particular concern is the now commonplace recommendation regarding how much fruit and vegetables we ought to be consuming. The issue is that, according to the logic of the Palaeolithic diets, more than 99% of our daily carbohydrates used to come from fruits and vegetables. For some of the year – and available only to some early human populations – honey would also have been included, but the overall contribution to the diet would have been close to negligible.

Nowadays fruits and vegetables have been forsaken so much as to become a rare snack or dessert food (in the case of fruit), with vegetables being more of a garnish with some meals rather than the bulk of carbohydrate. From this we can rightly deduce the carbohydrate source must have been replaced, and in our modern diets this tends to be mostly with cereal grains, some dairy and then refined carbohydrates (sugars contained in baked goods and snack foods). This has led to an exchange of nutrient-rich foods with alternatives that are less easily absorbed, much lower in micronutrient content, and higher in the sorts of fibres less beneficial than those in fruits and vegetables. These changes have been associated with poorer health of the gastrointestinal tract, challenges to acid-base balance within the blood, poor bone health, increased oxidative stress, increased rates of diabetes, arthritis, some cancers, cardiovascular disease and obesity.

The problem is not solely due to intakes of too few fruits and vegetables, because increasing intake of those will only help so much. The goal really should be to decrease our intakes of the alternatives, such as cereal-grain-foods, dairy and processed foods, and substitute those with fruits and vegetables. This should have the effect of maintaining a similar or slightly reduced total intake of carbohydrates, whilst increasing total intake of beneficial plant fibres and micronutrients, promoting the health of the gut, blood, bones and cells, and helping to protect against conditions associated with modern diets, such as diabetes, degenerative diseases, cardiovascular disease and obesity. At present, therefore, the current recommendations (such as '5 a day') are not really as helpful or conducive to good health as they need to be, because increasing fruit and vegetable intake on top of the normal diet, will not have as great an effect as replacing foods of little benefit with highly beneficial ones.

* * * * * * *

Fruits and vegetables are important for supporting the health of the immune system, although their effect is not immediate. A German study[14], assessed the effectiveness of tomato juice and carrot juice for improving immune function, and found that although the carotenoids reached the blood quite rapidly, the immune system was not improved until much later, with some factors responding best over a period of weeks. Other studies[15,16] have also shown that vegetables improve immune function, and that vegetables were better than fruits at improving the particular immune factors analysed.

The protective effects of fruits and vegetables are due to the wide spectrum of nutrients they contain, including various vitamins, minerals and any of thousands of other phytochemicals. These include groups such as carotenoids, flavonoids, tocopherols, lycopene, and others, as well as important dietary fibres. This in itself is the basis of one of many arguments against general multivitamin and mineral supplements for everyone, because although they will contain vitamins and minerals, they will not contain the thousands of other potentially beneficial nutrients found in whole foods.

Consuming fruits and vegetables throughout the day can lead to a constant flow of protective phytochemicals through the blood, which would not be the case on a minimal fruit and vegetable diet, supplemented with such a specific array of only a few, factory-processed nutrients. There can be a place for supplements, but a multi-vitamin/mineral pill should not be assumed to be an improvement to a diet rich in real foods, which would render such

51

supplements redundant, and potentially even harmful[*].

Further, we are still only in the early stages of understanding the actions specific phytochemicals actually have within the human body. For example, carotenoids and tocopherols contribute to vitamin activity and various other functions, such as antioxidant capacity, vision, supporting the immune system, and the healthy lifecycles of cells and tissues[17]. However, simply because a food might contain a rich source of a particular nutrient – such as vitamin C – this is not to say the health benefits derived from the food are necessarily a direct consequence of that particular nutrient[18]. For example, vitamin C might be thought of as particularly beneficial, because people who eat foods rich in vitamin C have been shown to be healthier than people who do not. But what if the benefit is not from vitamin C itself, but some other nutrient that happens to be in those foods as well, rendering the apparent benefits of vitamin C actually coincidental?

Nutrients do not tend to act alone, or confer benefits when taken in isolation, because they are involved in many processes with many other nutrients, and it is important to take plenty of nutrient-rich foods, rather than try to increase intake of particular ones, especially as they can be redundant without all the other nutrients to react with. Because phytochemicals occur in thousands of different types, it is not realistic to suppose researchers will have all of these – including all of their interactions and functions within the body – catalogued and fully described anytime soon.

Further, many important nutrients do not have a direct effect on health, but are involved in complex reactions in which the 'benefit' to health requires many other processes to be concurrently taking place. A particular phytochemical might not be protecting a cell from harm by itself, but be involved in complex reactions within the cell that support its function. It is often these secondary effects and

---

[*] Supplements are discussed in detail in their own chapter

interactions that are of greatest importance to overall health[18], but which happen to be most challenging to understand in terms of the health of individual cells.

One of the challenges to research concerning nutrients from fruits and vegetables, is that the relationship between the diet and what appears in the blood will vary according to various confounding variables. These could include body size, metabolic activity at a particular time of day, smoking, use of supplements, bioaccessibility and bioavailability, multiple sources of the nutrients, food processing and preparation techniques, times and temperatures, disease status[19] and the complexity of different foods consumed at the same time and in varying individual and combined amounts.

Raw versus Cooked Vegetables

As has already been discussed, certain nutrients, such as carotenoids, are better absorbed from cooked rather than raw vegetables[36], although anything that breaks the food up, such as chopping or pureeing, will increase availability of those nutrients. However, nutrients from different foods are affected by cooking in different ways and to differing extents. For example, sulforaphane – a chemical thought to be anti-carcinogenic – is more bioavailable from raw rather than cooked broccoli[37].

Over recent years a few books have been published on the subject of raw foods, which include recipes for smoothies and tout some of the benefits of raw vegetables. Whilst there certainly are benefits, it would be wrong to suppose that raw vegetables *in general* are healthier than cooked vegetables. Cooking helps break foods down, usually (but not always) making them more available for absorption through the gut. The main problem with eating a lot of raw vegetables is that this increases intake of phytic acid, which inhibits the absorption of certain essential nutrients.

Hence, although a few nutrients are better absorbed from raw foods, this can be at the expense of other, more important substances. With a general, mixed diet containing plenty of fresh fruit and vegetables, including some vegetables that are cooked and a few others raw, this is not an issue, as people will benefit from the best of all worlds. The problem arises when people become 'purist' in their approach, and so exclude cooked vegetables – this could potentially lead to mineral deficiencies that could present systemic challenges to the body. Decreasing mineral absorption could, for example, lead to an increased risk of osteoporosis, especially if raw vegetables are routinely consumed along with meats and fish, as these represent the most concentrated sources of many minerals and their absorption would be limited in the same way.

Perhaps one of the reasons for the increased interest in raw vegetables is connected to studies assessing the health benefits of such diets. For example, a recent study by a research group in the Netherlands[38], found that individuals with a high consumption of fruit and raw vegetables had the lowest risk of stroke. It could simply be that people who consume raw vegetables do so because they believe it is healthier, are interested in a healthy lifestyle, and therefore spend more time exercising, are less likely to smoke, and strive to eat more healthy foods in general. Considering that the phytochemicals associated with protection of blood vessels are better absorbed from cooked vegetables, there has to be more to it than that particular research paper reported. In any case, the study was sufficient to generate a need for us to improve our understanding of whatever underlying mechanisms might exist. Italian researchers[39] reported that raw red chicory presented both anti-oxidant and pro-oxidant activity[*], but the pro-oxidants were broken down during boiling whereas the anti-oxidants were not. Although this refers to only one type of vegetable, the message is simply that the issue is a complex one, and on balance the majority of benefits come with cooked rather than raw vegetables.

One warning against consuming raw vegetables is that plant foods from some parts of the world carry risk of infection from parasitic worms, and an association has been found between raw vegetable consumption and a particular type of meningitis in Taiwan[40], which involves the movement of worm larvae into the cerebrospinal fluid and brain. The parasite (Angiostrongylus cantonensis) can be found on plants and in snails, slugs, shrimp, crabs and prawns in Southeast Asia and around the Pacific. Any such foods from these regions should be cooked rather than consumed raw.

Taking this a step further, a Korean study[41] recently published a report on raw vegetable juice. Their finding was that a commercially available raw vegetable juice increased risks of acquiring harmful bacteria, fungi and parasites. However, irradiating the juice not only made the product safer, but increased its anti-oxidant potential too.

* * * * * * *

Soil can be contaminated by the use of fertilizers, pesticides, contaminated wastewater and other sources of industrial and domestic waste. These contaminants can then become the substance of whatever is grown from such affected soil. British investigators[45]

---

[*] Discussed in chapter on Oxidative and Nitrosative Stress

recently published a report on the presence of certain metals in vegetables, and noted that concentrations varied between plant types. Exposure to contaminated vegetables can best be reduced by purchasing organically-grown vegetables or growing vegetables at home. Alternatively, varying the types of vegetables consumed from day to day and week to week will help reduce exposure to any one contaminant, which should permit the body to recover between exposures, reducing any risk of actual harm.

Increasing Fruit & Vegetable Intake

One of the greatest problems for individual health is the lack of sufficient fruits and vegetables within the diet. In a recent American study[46], and an earlier joint European and American study[23], it was found that people were consuming less than the recommended five servings of fruit and vegetables a day, in spite of direct recommendations and strategies to increase intake in these individuals. However, it was found that consuming a commercially-available vegetable juice each day was sufficient to bridge the gap. Further, vegetable juice intake has been demonstrated to be an effective means of reducing oxidative damage to DNA[47], which is important for cancer prevention. Another study showed that vegetable juice and tomato soup were both effective at reducing oxidative damage to cholesterol[48], which is beneficial for cardiovascular health.

Importantly, health promoters should place less emphasis on recommending only an increase in fruit and vegetable intake, as this might wrongly be construed as a necessity to eat more food overall. Rather, the focus should be on the substitution of less beneficial sources of carbohydrates, with healthier fruits and vegetables. This needs to be a gradual approach, where improvements are made to individual meals, rather than an attempt to overhaul the diet in one go, which would be more challenging, less reasonable and less realistic.

Digestibility and Absorption

"No diet will remove all the fat from your body because the brain is entirely fat. Without a brain, you might look good, but all you could do is run for public office."

- George Bernard Shaw

How various phytochemicals are digested and absorbed is still being investigated[20,21], and assessment techniques are continually being improved upon[22]. The finer details of bioaccessibility and bioavailability are complicated to assess in humans during normal life, where foods are eaten in combinations and it is difficult to assess what appears in the blood from food, and what appears there from cells and organs.

Carotenoids give fruits and vegetables their colour, and have been associated with the powerful antioxidant properties of these foods. However, there are various types of carotenoids, with different properties and different specific effects, and their concentrations within different fruits and vegetables will vary according to the type of carotenoid, species of plant, size of the food and its ripeness. Absorption of carotenoids into the blood requires them to have been sufficiently broken down during digestion. Further, although carotenoids such as beta-carotene are potent defenders against oxidative damage*, they do not work alone and require numerous anti-oxidant factors to be present in order to confer benefits[23].

A study by French investigators[24], reported on how the stomach is important for transferring carotenoids from within the cells

---

* Discussed further in chapter on Oxidative and Nitrosative Stress

of the plant food into fats which can later transport the nutrients in the blood. Different carotenoids compete with each other; meaning more of certain ones are absorbed with each meal[24]. Further, although carotenoids are damaged by heating at and above the temperatures involved in sterilisation, they are unharmed during pasteurisation and boiling[25], meaning that commercially available fruit and vegetable juices can be useful sources of these nutrients.

In an assessment of the bioavailability of vitamin C from various sources, it was found that this was roughly equivalent in whole orange sections, orange juice, vitamin C tablets (with and without iron) and cooked broccoli[26]. The bioavailability of vitamin C was 20% lower in raw broccoli, although it was concluded this would have little negative impact in a diet containing various sources of vitamin C[26]. These findings, including that cooked broccoli is a slightly better source of vitamin C than raw broccoli, was supported by another, similar study[27].

Boiling, grilling, microwave-cooking and steaming have all been shown to decrease the beta-carotene content of vegetables equally, although what remained was better able to be absorbed than from raw vegetables, and increased blood content to a greater extent than from the raw foods[28]. The total carotenoid content of vegetables differs significantly between individual and mixed vegetables, and how well these are absorbed will vary according to the presence of additional fats and fibres with the meal[29].

Vegetable oil, oat bran and wheat bran decrease the potential for nutrient absorption, whilst olive oil, peanut oil and rapeseed oil improve absorption potential[29]. Some fat needs to be present in the stomach when vegetables are being broken down, as fat-soluble nutrients, such as the carotenoids, tocopherols and some vitamins, need to be transported with fats into the blood[21,24]. However, the total amount of fat required is very low (3-5 grams per meal)[21].

A recent study by British investigators[30] found that the intact cell walls of vegetables were sufficient to prevent carotene moving from within those cells through the gut wall and into the blood. Hence, although chewing food and the other digestive processes are important for promoting absorption of nutrients, the greater the level of chopping and even pureeing of vegetables, the greater the availability of the nutrients becomes, as these help break up the cells and make the nutrients more bioaccessible. This suggests particular benefits of juice smoothies and vegetable soups.

Another study[31], reported that vegetable juice (having been pureed and heated) was a better source of alpha-carotene and lutein than raw or cooked whole vegetables. The authors concluded that the pureeing caused more damage to the individual vegetable cells, which made the nutrients more available for absorption in the gut. However, levels of three other nutrients tested (beta-carotene, beta-cryptoxanthin and lycopene) did not differ between groups (pureed and heated, whole raw or whole cooked)[31]. It was commented on that non-pureed fruits and vegetables reduce absorption of nutrients because of their fibre content (which is broken down during pureeing). However, as fibre is particularly important for human health this helps illustrate the point that variety is key, with different benefits of whole foods and pureed ones, and it would be useful to include both in the diet.

In addition to how vegetables are prepared, there are of course differences between the nutrient contents of different vegetables. However, it is not sufficient to know which foods have the greatest concentration of whichever nutrient, because what we really want to know is which foods provide the greatest concentration of that nutrient to the blood.

Researchers in the Netherlands[32] reported that although spinach contains ten times more beta-carotene than broccoli and green peas, consumption of spinach led to no detectable increase in blood beta-carotene concentrations, whereas they increased significantly following ingestion of broccoli and green peas. As it happens, although spinach is rich in many useful nutrients, absorption of nutrients from spinach is very, very poor, rendering it a fairly useless food for humans (other animals may have different relationships with spinach, but as we are not them we would do better to prefer broccoli and other vegetables).

Overall, fruit has been found to be far more effective than green leafy vegetables at increasing blood levels of vitamin A, but variations between the bioavailability of fruits (21-100%) and green, leafy vegetables (8-46%) are further exacerbated by differences between people[33]. Other vegetables may contribute more vitamin A than the green, leafy vegetables, but in any case the greatest source of this vitamin is from organ meats, particularly liver (liver is not recommended for pregnant women, as the concentrations of vitamin A can be so high they represent a risk to foetal development).

Vitamin A is beneficial for supporting the normal health and functioning of the eyes. Lutein is an important carotenoid that could also be particularly beneficial for eye health, and has been shown to be five times more bioavailable from vegetables than beta-carotene[11]. Overall, eye health – as just one example – is best supported by including in the diet a variety of fruits, vegetables and organ meats, which provide beta-carotene, lutein, vitamin A and many other important nutrients, all in differing concentrations and bioavailabilities.

How crops are harvested and processed can have effects on carotenoid concentration and bioavailability of foods[35]. Because of this there are now emerging trends in agriculture to promote the health benefits to be conferred from crops. This should not seem unusual, as the recent increase in 'organic' foods followed consumer demand for plant foods with fewer and less chemicals used in their production. It is worth pointing out, however, that 'organic' certainly does not mean 'chemical-free', but simply that there are regulations in place to ensure that to categorise a food as organic certain requirements must be met. These requirements vary considerably from country to country, and really the only way to ensure foods are chemical-free is to grow them at home using organic compost and soil. Despite this, the agricultural sciences are researching how to most effectively increase the nutritional benefits of farmed foods.

Bioaccessibility & Bioavailability

"The foods that promote longevity, virtue, strength, health,
happiness, and joy; are juicy, smooth, substantial,
and agreeable to the stomach."

- Bhagavad Gita

The properties of foods will differ between and within species. The age, health and diet of a food source will affect its chemical composition to some extent. As animals age their meat is likely to contain more fat, and as plant foods ripen they can increase their concentration of certain sugars and other nutrients. Processing and cooking of foods can alter the food's nutrient content and how effectively those nutrients are absorbed across the gut into the blood. Because this varies between nutrients within the same foods, between different foods, and between cooking and processing methods, it is unrealistic to give specific details about all foods and nutrients, other than in a few key examples as we go.

In the mouth, the chewing of food helps to break it down mechanically, whilst enzymes in saliva break it down chemically. In the stomach the mechanical and chemical breakdown of food continues, as the stomach contracts and imparts compressive forces on foods to promote their digestion. The gastric fluid can disintegrate the food from the outside, and the movement of food particles against each other causes friction and shear stresses[49], causing it to break up and expose a larger surface area to enzymes and stomach acid.

As foods are broken open in the stomach, the contents of cells mix with the gastric juice. This chiefly affects fats, proteins, vitamins, minerals and phytochemicals. How effectively this happens can be further affected by the total amount of food ingested, the presence of additional fluid, temperature, pH, time, viscosity and the agitation caused by stomach contractions[49]. In difference to the food types mentioned above, carbohydrates and their constituents are largely broken down in the mouth and gut, rather than the stomach. This is due to the enzymes in the mouth and gut being more specialised at breaking down carbohydrates than those in the stomach[10].

The *bioaccessibility* of a substance refers to how much of it is present in the gut, and this is determined by the amount liberated from within the original foodstuff during digestion[10]. For example, a vitamin supplement might have a high content of vitamin E, but if the pill is not broken down during digestion, it will pass through the digestive tract with none of the vitamin E being liberated. Hence, the vitamin E content of the supplement would be high, but it would not be bioaccessible. The key to producing a good supplement or drug is to ensure the pill breaks up in the right part of the digestive tract: too early and the nutrients might be destroyed, too late and they might not be absorbed into the blood.

Bioavailability, on the other hand, refers to the amount of a nutrient that is available to the body for physiological processes or storage. So, perhaps we now have a supplement containing highly bioaccessible vitamin E, meaning that the vitamin is liberated from the pill in the right way. Because vitamin E needs to be bonded onto fat for digestion, and the pill was a solid tablet rather than an oil-filled one, the vitamin E is not absorbed into the blood unless taken with an additional source of fat. Hence, something can be highly bioaccessible but not bioavailable. Alternatively, because the nutrient was manufactured synthetically in a laboratory, it might not be used by the body, as its natural alternative would be, perhaps rendering it useless.   Again, this could be described as being of poor bioavailability.

Some nutrients, such as beta-carotene in fruits and vegetables, are reduced in certain foods during cooking, but can become better absorbed as a result, whereas beta-carotene in other foods can become reduced and less absorbable due to cooking. Although this raises questions about which foods should or should not be heated to promote the bioavailability of beta-carotene, other carotenoids and many other important nutrients become more bioavailable once they are cooked.   The result is that we can recommend a variety of foods, prepared in a variety of ways, with different benefits from each. Further, we ought to be sceptical about food labels listing nutritional composition, as the total amounts included will almost certainly not be what is both bioaccessible and bioavailable. This is true whether the food is a breakfast cereal with synthetic vitamins and minerals added, a supplement, or a fruit or vegetable.

Proteins

"If we could give every individual the right amount of nourishment and exercise, not too little and not too much, we would have found the safest way to health."

- Hippocrates

Proteins are the building blocks of life, made from strands of amino acids. The blueprint of the human body is contained within our DNA. That DNA is housed within the nucleus of each cell, and its function is to pass parts of its code over to other areas within the cell, where amino acids can be made into new strands, and ultimately form new proteins. These might be structural components of the cell, or enzymes required for catalysing reactions. Whether they are muscle cells, nerve cells, blood cells, the structural framework of bones or the enzymes involved in every aspect of our biological processes, proteins are a fundamental nutrient for animal life on Earth.

Dietary proteins are broken down in the stomach and metabolised in the liver, from where the amino acids can then be transported in the blood and taken up by cells where they are needed, whether as structural components based upon the DNA code, or else converted into energy. Any excess amino acids are broken down further, with some components recycled and others eliminated in the urine. If there are insufficient proteins in the diet, then proteins already within tissues of the body can be broken down, although as energy mostly comes from fats and carbohydrates, so protein losses in these circumstances are usually minimal. Proteins can be broken down for energy preferentially during fasting/starvation, as the body alters its metabolism to preserve its fat stores.

Because of the availability of modern foods, it is straightforward enough for individuals to be vegetarian and to obtain all the protein they require from plant foods. However, that protein has to come from cereal grains, dairy products, beans, seeds and legumes, which are not ideal sources. The proteins in legumes, for example, limit the absorption of important nutrients, including minerals such as iron, so there can be compromises. Further, none of these foods are well digested by the human gut.

It is commonly argued that proteins from plants are not as bioavailable as those from animal source foods[50], and this is true, but the difference is typically so minimal that it is not really an argument against plant proteins. The benefit of animal source foods is not just that they are more bioavailable, but rather that they can be better assimilated into structural components, due to the similarity between the proteins in animal meats and proteins in our own body. However, it is not only their protein content that makes animal source foods of great value to us.

Animal foods (including fish) are our most important source of bioavailable minerals and essential fatty acids. As already discussed, the mineral content of modern vegetables is not readily bioavailable due to the presence of phytic acid, and instead the greatest value of these foods is in their content of fibres, vitamins, and phytochemicals, including carotenes, flavonoids, and luteins. Our best sources of minerals and essential fatty acids are animals and fish. Although the same minerals and some essential fats can be found in vegetarian foods, they are not as useable by the body, so in some cases it would be preferable for vegetarians to supplement their diet with these where there is risk of deficiencies.

A relatively high protein intake is also associated with more favourable blood cholesterol levels and improved insulin sensitivity, and these effects are particularly noted when a high carbohydrate diet is exchanged for one with approximately equal amounts of carbohydrates and proteins (35% of each)[51]. Research has also demonstrated that a high intake of proteins is associated with a reduced risk of certain cardiovascular risk factors and types of stroke[52,53], although some related findings are still disputed[54]. With proteins and carbohydrates contributing almost equally to the diet, the remainder should be made up of mostly unsaturated fats[*].

One concern with high protein intakes is a *potentially* negative effect on the pH levels of the blood, because proteins might have an acidifying effect (demonstrating this in the blood is problematic because acids are rapidly buffered[†]). Because bones are a storage site for minerals, and some of those minerals are involved in maintaining a balanced blood acid-base balance, there has been much research into the effects of proteins on bone health. This is a fairly detailed and important topic, and so it is dealt with in its own chapter later on. Suffice it to state our Palaeolithic ancestors – with their relatively high protein intakes – actually had far more robust bones than we have, and this has been attributed to the importance of proteins for bone health, the acid-buffering capacity of fruits and vegetables, and the high levels of bone-strengthening physical activity.

Some sources of protein increase the amount of sulphur in the gut, which has been linked to inflammatory bowel disease (IBD), due to its harmful effects on the protective lining of the intestines. The main culprits are the preservatives found in some meats (nitrates), which have been banned from just about everything else, but have been allowed to persist in sausages, bacon, salami and so on.

Other foods to avoid in excess due to their sulphur content include eggs and red meat, although an excessive intake of red meat

---

[*] Discussed in the chapter on Fats
[†] Discussed in the chapter on Acid-Base Balance

should be avoided for other reasons besides gut health alone. Sulphur in the gut can also be increased from dairy foods, beer and some other alcoholic drinks, breads and fish. Out of all of these, red meats and fish are the only ones we would have experienced during our evolutionary pasts. A moderate intake is unlikely to cause harm, and we need only concern ourselves with avoiding high intakes of these foods, particularly the processed meats. It is noteworthy that inflammatory bowel disease is also promoted by stress, and prevented by a high intake of vegetable-derived fibres, certain anti-oxidants and physical activity.

* * * * * * *

The main challenge for vegetarians is in obtaining sufficient plant proteins, whilst avoiding foods that are less beneficial, such as cereal grains and dairy products. Animal proteins should come from a variety of meats and fish, and should not be overcooked[*]. A high intake of red meat and preserved meats is associated with an increased risk of certain cancers.

Further, the animal foods to be included in the diet should be more than just the meat itself, and include the nutrient-richer organ meats too. Poultry should also be included, as well as fish and to a lesser extent eggs. Substituting a high carbohydrate diet for one approximately equal in its content of protein and carbohydrate has been found to have beneficial effects on cardiovascular health, including a preferred blood cholesterol profile and reduced risk of certain types of stroke.

---

[*] Discussed in the chapter on Red Meat and Cancer

Meat

"If there hadn't been women we'd still be squatting in a cave eating raw meat, because we made civilization in order to impress our girlfriends."

- Orson Welles

From an evolutionary perspective, we know that animal source foods were the defining feature in the development of larger brains, shorter guts, tool development and persistence of bipedal locomotion. Because this has been covered in *Human Evolution, Diet and Health*, it does not make sense to revisit all the details here. In brief, gorillas consume a diet high in relatively energy-poor and fibrous plant foods, with some insects, and spend a large portion of their day in the same place, investing most of their time eating. Chimpanzees, by contrast, consume more meat, more insects and more fruit, and spend more of their day actively moving about and foraging. Humans, historically at least, were the most active ape. Family groups would likely have been divided into those members who gathered fruits and tubers, and those who hunted.

In addition to the finds of cutting tools developed for removing meat from bones, we have remains of animal bones with stone tool cut marks on them, bones split open so the bone marrow could be accessed, and brain cases holed-out so the contents could be gotten at too. In fact, where most animals would have had to leave the bone marrow and brain because they were so hard to access, our ingenuity permitted us to access them after the big cats had left them alone. This is particularly noteworthy, because the bone marrow and brain were the organs with the highest concentrations of omega-3 fatty acids[*].

One concern we have nowadays is the association between red meat consumption and cancers. This will be discussed in greater detail in the next chapter, but it is important to appreciate that the dangers are associated with products of cooked meat, rather than raw. Although it is difficult to ascertain when we regularly began cooking food, it would not have been until relatively recently, in an evolutionary sense at least. Establishing when is complicated, because although there is evidence of fires at ancient human settlements, there are few where charred bones have been found, which would indicate the cooking of foods. Even then it is difficult to know if this would have been an isolated group and how often food would have been cooked.

Most carnivores in the wild prefer to consume organs meats and the digestive tracts of their prey animals first, with the actual meat being left until last or for the subordinates. Although the meat is a rich source of highly bioavailable protein, with some useful fats, vitamins and minerals, the organ meats are far more nutritionally dense, at least in terms of the micronutrient profiles.

That red meat is now so popular is a product of more recent trends and habits, rather than an evolutionary clinger-on. In fact, our preference as a society to avoid organ meats actually makes fish a far healthier alternative, as the fatty acid profile is richer and more concentrated than what we can derive from meat alone. As we shall see, the most suitable recommendation may be to include a variety of meats, organ meats and fish in the weekly diet, rather than focus on any one of these in isolation.

A high consumption of meat has been hypothesised to increase bone turnover (as discussed in the chapter on bone health).

---

[*] The omega-3 fatty acids are discussed in the chapter on fats.

One study[326] which compared a diet comprising six servings of meat a week with a high carbohydrate diet actually reported increased bone turnover in the high carbohydrate group, and concluded that the low-sodium, net-base (alkali) diet in the high meat group was responsible for protecting bones. An optimal bone health requires a sufficient intake of protein, an overall pH-neutral diet including a low-sodium intake, and sufficient physical activity. It is important to state, however, that this does not refer to a diet high in alkaline foods, but one with a combination of foods in which the beneficial proteins are buffered by base-producing fruits and vegetables, as will be discussed in greater detail in the respective chapters.

When pooled together, total red and processed meat intakes have been associated with increased risk of a sub-category of stroke (cerebral infarction), but not other types of stroke[55]. However, when fresh meat intake was assessed independently of processed meat, there was no risk of any kind of stroke[55]. As discussed in the previous chapter, a high protein intake is actually protective against certain types of stroke and can promote cardiovascular health. It is therefore important not to regard all this as giving mixed messages. Unprocessed red meat might not be a risk factor for stroke, but it remains a risk for certain types of cancers. A higher red meat intake has also been associated with metabolic syndrome and central obesity in individuals at risk of cardiovascular disease[56], but the evidence is conflicting and weak[57]. In terms of cardiovascular health, a high protein intake should include proteins from all foods, including poultry and fish.

A recent study[58] has shown that red meat from animals reared on grass is higher in omega-3 fats, than that of animals receiving a food concentrate used in some feeds. Although the authors of that study concluded this would be of benefit to people who normally eat red meat, it is still appropriate to avoid eating red meat too often, and to find other ways of increasing dietary omega-3 intake.

Interestingly, chickens fed a diet rich in polyunsaturated fats had lower body fat levels than chickens consuming equivalent amounts of saturated fats[59]. The diets of the animals we eat can have a direct effect on our own health, both in terms of total fat composition and the type of fat. It seems that a more natural approach to diet is important for those animals too, and the benefits are passed on to us as consumers.

In contrast to the positive influences of a natural diet on animal health, and consequently our own health, many of us are aware there might be problems with the administration of growth promoters to animals. We can be exposed to these substances ourselves following consumption of the meat, which can subsequently disrupt our own hormone balance. A recent study[60] conducted by a group in the U.S. and published in 2011, reported the presence of oestrone and progesterone in chicken litter, amongst other hormone disrupters. The use of hormones to promote the growth of lean muscle in cattle has been banned in Europe[61], although reports have shown that the illicit use of such hormones still persists. Part of the problem lies in detection of abnormal hormone levels in animals, which could be useful not only for establishing the likelihood that an animal has received a growth promoter, but for monitoring normal health too. The challenge has been in establishing what normal hormone levels are in animals, and despite much research attention, there is still relatively little definitive data[62].

Another serious concern is the use of antibiotics in animals, as these can also act as growth promoters, and have been used for this purpose since the 1940s. There are three potential problems associated with these antibiotics. Firstly, humans could potentially be at risk of allergic or other reactions to the antibiotics, although such risks are negligible[63]. Secondly, by exposure to any antibiotic-resistant bacteria, those bacteria might be transferred to the human gut[64]. Thirdly, long-term exposure to the antibiotics within meat could cause our own bacteria to develop resistance[63]. A recent study by an Italian group[64] published in 2011, demonstrated that certain bacterial species in the digestive systems of chicken and pigs have become resistant to antibiotics, and that these traits can then transfer to us.

Let us suppose there are thousands of different species of bacteria within the gut of a chicken, and there are millions of bacteria of each species. Over time, because bacteria increase in numbers at such a fast rate, there are plenty of genetic mutations that occur. Mostly mutations tend to quickly kill-off an individual organism, although sometimes they actually do no harm and the organism has a normal life. In very rare occasions there is actually some benefit of the mutation. If that benefit is such that the organism stands a better chance of reproducing than others, then over time that genetic mutation spreads amongst the descendents, replacing the previous and less beneficial 'norm'.

So, in a gut that is being bombarded by antibiotics – which have the effect of killing off many bacteria – it is quite reasonable to suppose that out of the millions upon millions of rapidly reproducing bacteria, some will be more resistant to antibiotics than others. Over time, that new level of resistance will become the norm, until a stronger level of resistance develops, even better at withstanding the antibiotics than the previous. Soon enough, that particular type of antibiotic is rendered entirely ineffectual, and so new ones are introduced. This has been going on since the 1940s, with plenty of different antibiotics and many different species of bacteria evolving, many carrying similar genetic mutations that have given them resistance to whatever they are presented with. Regardless of whether the initial reason for administering the antibiotic was for growth promotion or to prevent or treat an infection, the consequences are the same. When transferred to us, we have a reduced ability to respond to those antibiotics too, which could have serious repercussions should we require them for the treatment of a serious infection.

The problem is that the genes carrying the mutation can be transferred to the bacteria within our own guts, when the bacteria from the animals meet our own stock[64,65]. Our exposure to those bacteria and genes is not only through direct contact with the meat. The faeces of those animals are comprised in large proportion of bacteria, the growth promoting antibiotics and other hormone disrupters. From animal waste-removal practices those substances are transferred to the soil, and can ultimately end up in drinking water and foods, including vegetables[65]. Another recent study[66] published in 2011 by a Swiss research group, reported that (with one exception) more than 54% of the bacterial strains they analysed were resistant to a variety of antibiotics. Their sample population, from which those antibiotic-resistant bacteria were assessed, comprised cows, calves, veterinarians and pig farmers. The same study[66], reported antibiotic resistance in just over a quarter of strains taken from minced meat, tank milk, pigs and slaughterhouse employees. Their samples were collected as recently as 2009.

This poses a real threat to human health, and as a result the World Health Organisation (WHO) and the Economic and Social Committee of the European Union have both decided this is a public health issue[63]. The bans that have been put in place as a consequence of this can be expected to reduce (but not eliminate) the total quantities of antibiotics administered to animals.

One complication is that reducing the use of antibiotics as growth promoters increases the amount of infections in animals, meaning they have to be administered antibiotics for therapeutic reasons. However, the overall result is a general reduction in the total amount of antibiotics we now have in our food. Considering this situation has been developing since the 1940s, it has been the bans of the late 1990s – based upon convincing scientific research – which have led to the greater awareness of the problems associated with antibiotics, and the overall reduction in their use over the last decade or so. Most importantly, the increased risks of infection from resistant bacteria or viral strains being transferred from infected birds and animals to us, is expected to support an ever-decreasing use of antibiotics in animals.

It has been a natural consequence of our demands on society that food has been tampered with as it has. We want society to support our growing population and ensure we have sufficient food for everyone, and so pressures are increasing for farmers to produce more food from animals that are heavier, taste better, and remain in good health until slaughter. Despite these pressures for ever-increasing efficiency, it would be very wrong to assume that matters only become worse, with our own health always being sacrificed as a consequence.

Agricultural scientists face an incredible challenge, whereby the expectation is that so much food is produced, despite increased risks of serious infections spreading amongst ever-increasing animal groups, and that costs of meat production are kept low. What is particularly important is the awareness of how human health must be protected, so much so that not only are the agricultural scientists interested in limiting antibiotic use, but they are also focussed on improving food quality, such as by augmenting diets of animals to increase the omega-3 fat content of the meat. It would be a depressing reflection upon modern times if we only saw the doom and gloom, at the expense of seeing how improvements are being made, and will continue to be made. The gap between the average of what is offered, and what is optimal for our own health, then comes down to personal decision-making, whereby we can choose to source meat from animals not exposed to growth promoters.

Whilst attempting to keep a positive spin from the science and technology front, it is important to state research is not only being used to improve how healthy meat can be, but to ensure eating pleasure is maximised too. A research group made up of investigators from Scotland and Italy[67], assessed genetic traits of Aberdeen Angus beef cattle, in order to identify which traits were associated with the tenderness, density and smell of the meat. The purpose of that study was to help ensure that the cattle with those particular genes were selected for mating, because genetic testing can obviously be conducted during life, whereas meat quality cannot otherwise be assessed until it is too late for the owner to perpetuate such traits.

* * * * * * *

One of the biggest challenges faced by researchers investigating the health consequences of certain foods, is the matter of confounding variables. A study published in 2009[57] reported that those consuming the highest amount of red meat were predisposed to increased levels of inflammation and had poor blood cholesterol concentrations. However, it was also noted that those who consumed the most red meat were the least physically active, were heaviest and had the highest waist circumference, whereas those who ate the least red meat also consumed the fewest calories overall, with low intakes of fat, protein, cholesterol and vegetable oils, and had higher intakes of fibre, fruits, vegetables, white meat and fish. So, is it appropriate to conclude red meat predisposes people to inflammation and high cholesterol levels, or that these factors were caused by low intakes of fruits, vegetables and oily fish, and exacerbated by insufficient levels of physical activity? As the study did not try to analyse these differences further it is difficult for us to know. However, it is reasonable to suppose an unhealthy lifestyle and diet deficient in fruits, vegetables and essential fats is most likely to have negative health consequences, when compared to a more physically active lifestyle that includes a variety of good foods.

* * * * * * *

To state that a vegetarian diet is healthier than a diet which includes meat is certainly not true, and there is no good quality evidence to support such an idea. If we were to compare vegetarians with people who eat mostly fish, poultry, fresh fruits and vegetables, there is every reason to suppose the vegetarians would do less well, depending upon which aspects of health we are assessing. Consuming three meals or more each week of red meat, or red meat that has been overcooked or charred, or exposed to high temperatures during cooking, is associated with increased risk of developing certain cancers (as discussed in the next chapter). There have also been associations between meat intake and heart disease, but then the research has demonstrated that substituting saturated fats for carbohydrates actually worsens cholesterol levels, which is indicative of a greater risk to cardiovascular health. It is not an issue of vegetarianism compared to meat eating, but rather an issue of how to have a healthy diet, comprised of various foods that do us good, prepared most often in a healthy way.

Foods high in saturated fats should be substituted for foods rich in essential fats and proteins. Red meat consumption should be limited to twice a week or less, and it should be cooked at low temperatures for as short a period of time as appropriate to make the food safe. To state that because too much red meat is bad, therefore all meat is bad and vegetarianism is the obvious alternative is not a sensible or logical argument. It is certainly no different to suggesting that because a very high carbohydrate intake is potentially harmful to cardiovascular health, therefore everybody should limit their intake of fruits and vegetables. Meats and organ meats contain many important fats, vitamins and minerals. Vegetarians can acquire all the protein they need from vegetarian sources, although to do so may encourage problems with gut health and promote nutrient deficiencies unless supplemented for (particularly fat-soluble nutrients, some minerals, and some essential fatty acids, which have poor bioavailability when from vegetarian sources).

This is really not supposed to be some anti-vegetarian crusade, but rather it is to illustrate the point that vegetarianism is not a perfect diet, nor is it a natural one for human beings, but then again neither is a diet containing cooked meat (although raw meat must definitely be avoided nowadays). There have to be compromises with any approach, but people should choose vegetarianism for personal reasons, not because of a belief that it is the healthiest approach. There are issues with meat consumption, but the solution is to be careful about how meat contributes to the diet, not to exclude it entirely.

Red Meat & Cancer

"Heaven sends us good meat, but the devil sends cooks."
- David Garrick

The consumption of red and processed meats has been associated with an increased risk of certain cancers, including prostate[68], oesophageal and gastric cancers[12,69]. However, the underlying mechanisms are not yet fully understood. Some studies[69] have reported an association between the content of heme-iron and heterocyclic amines (to be discussed in this chapter), whilst others have associated the risk with increased nitrite consumption[12].

Heterocyclic Aromatic Amines

Heterocyclic aromatic amines (HAAs) are a collection of chemicals produced when meats are cooked. The formation of some of these has been associated with damage to the genetic material within cells, in turn leading to gene mutations. Genes are coded messages for how a cell should behave (what it does, how it develops and when it should be expected to die so it can be replaced). Should a critically important gene be altered, and should that mutation cause too much cell material to be produced (by interfering with a 'stop' signal), there is a risk of cancer development. That such substances are formed in cooked meats is well established in the scientific literature[70,71], and individuals who consume red meat on a daily basis are thereby regularly exposed to these carcinogens.

However, the actual risk from one isolated gene within one isolated cell, following exposure to a single meal is negligible. In any case, the immune system should identify the unusual cell and destroy it. A problem arises if many carcinogens are consumed regularly and over an extended period, meaning that at some point a cancerous cell is not destroyed, and a risk for proliferation exists that can ultimately lead to far more serious consequences. It is not only important to determine which foods increase risk and how, but we should also have an awareness of which foods are protective. By knowing more about these we can better look after ourselves, so as to promote our health rather than compromise it.

A recent review[72] found no association between cancer risk and the dietary intake of heterocyclic aromatic amines formed in meats during cooking. This is not because HAAs are not carcinogenic, but rather that they are typically consumed with other natural substances in food that are protective against cancers. So, with a specific cancer affecting only a small percentage of the population, and there being so many potential risk factors, studies need to have thousands of subjects in order to establish whether or not a single food can really make a significant difference to risk. However, an English research team[71] recently established a mechanism whereby a particular chemical from cooked meats could affect the brain's pituitary gland and disrupt normal hormone activity. These mechanisms were proposed as a potential pathway for how that chemical in cooked meat could increase the risk of breast cancer.

Another problem with cooking meats (and fish) is that the fats become heated and undergo chemical changes as a consequence. Even if the fats are not overcooked, the stomach can increase the amount of damage caused to them from partial heating, increasing the risk of absorbing potentially harmful fats into the blood[73]. The accumulation of harmful fats has been associated with an increased risk not only of cancers, but of diabetes and heart disease too[73].

Red Meat & Breast Cancer

Hormones act within the body as chemical messengers, travelling in the blood all around the body, either free or linked onto a protein that carries them around. A hormone will not work on every cell in the body, because only certain cells will have 'receptors' for it, and the hormone will have to bind onto that receptor before its message can be passed into the cell. Breast cancers can be categorised according to whether or not these receptors are involved in the cancer development, so there are hormone receptor-positive and hormone receptor-negative cancers. With breast cancer, the hormones most likely to be involved are the female sex hormones: the oestrogens and progesterone.

An American research group[74] assessed data collected from 90,659 women over 12 years, of whom 1,021 reported cases of breast cancer. The authors of that study concluded there was a strong, positive association between red meat intake and hormone receptor-positive breast cancers, but not hormone receptor-negative ones, for both oestrogens and progesterone. Importantly, the authors assessed potentially confounding variables, such as fruit and vegetable intake, and found that the risk was between red meat itself and cancer development. Further, the association was related to the number of grams consumed, rather than servings, implying that the risk is due to the total amount rather than how often red meat is eaten.

From that research paper[74], it was clear that processed meats, hot dogs and bacon all carry an increased risk of breast cancer development, but unprocessed beef and pork were associated with breast cancers too. The authors concluded the underlying mechanism for cancer development could be related to hormonal pathways, which is supported by the findings of the previously mentioned study on heterocyclic amines from cooked meats[71]. There is a potential for growth promoters to increase hormone-related cancer risk as well, although there were no studies available which had assessed this specifically, and the current ban in effect in Europe should at least reduce exposure of Europeans to this potential source of cancer development.

One American study[75] assessed the red meat intake and breast cancer risk amongst 39,268 pre-menopausal women, and found those who consumed the highest amounts of red meat during adolescence were at a 30-40% higher risk of developing breast cancer than those with the lowest intakes. They noted that risk increased by 20% for every additional 100 grams of daily red meat consumption. As with the study by the other American group[74], the association was strongest for the hormone-receptor positive cancers. Interestingly, they found that adult red meat intake was not significantly associated with risk of breast cancer in that group.

The researchers also noted that women who consumed the highest amounts of red meat during adolescence were also most likely to be current smokers, have higher body weight and calorie intake, and to have gained the most weight during adulthood. Understanding the underlying mechanisms of why this should be is interesting, but not within the scope of this book to investigate further. Was a high red meat intake associated* with a predisposition to other less healthy lifestyle factors (such as smoking, being overweight, etc.), or could it be that the effects of red meat on hormones is the underlying cause of these behavioural changes? Further, is this for any red meat, for

---

* It is important not to interpret an association as cause and effect, as it is often not possible to know which is which

processed red meats, overcooked meats or meats with the highest composition of hormone-disrupting chemicals?

Red Meat & Colorectal Cancer

A study published in 2010[76] compared diets and prevalence of colorectal cancer amongst whites and African Americans. They found that total protein intake was associated with a risk reduction for colorectal cancer, with the effect being stronger for whites than African Americans. The authors suggested that fresh meat might reduce risk, whereas processed meat could elevate it, as only processed meat showed any significantly increased risk of those types of cancer. These findings are in agreement with a meta-analysis performed in 2011[77], which concluded there was insufficient evidence to support a link between red meat intake and colorectal cancer. One suggestion in that paper was that confounding variables might have been responsible for any apparent relationships between dietary red meat and colorectal cancer[77].

In contrast to the findings of those investigations, others have found a positive association. An investigation by a Canadian group[78] compared colorectal cancer risk with total red meat intake, cooking methods and levels of doneness, and particular genetic factors. They found that red meat consumption above two servings a week increased risk, and that genetic factors did not interact with overall red meat consumption to influence that risk. Interestingly, however, certain genetic factors did increase the risk of colorectal cancer more than four-fold in those with the highest intake of *well-done* red meat. So, a high intake increased risk, and a high intake of well-done red meat increased risk further in those with a particular genetic trait. An increased risk of some cancers has certainly been associated with genetic predisposition, but this has not been found to be the case with all cancers, including colorectal cancer and prostate cancer[68], unless overcooked.

Disappointingly, although the authors of the Canadian study[78] did assess fruit and vegetable intake, in addition to other dietary and lifestyle factors, these were not mentioned in their results, making it difficult for the reader to see that any confounding variables were taken into account. Low numbers of subjects, in both this study and others in which no association was found, make it difficult to draw definitive conclusions.

In agreement with the study by the Canadian group[78], an American group[79] also reported an association between red meat intake and colorectal cancer risk, and noted that risk was higher for individuals with a particular genetic trait who consumed a high amount of well-done meat. These researchers stated that fruit and vegetable intake did not significantly reduce risk of colorectal cancer, although there was a lack of detail in the study and other lifestyle factors were not mentioned (it would be interesting to establish whether a high fibre intake was protective, as was reported in a rat study[80]). The American researchers concluded that red meat should not be consumed three times a week or more, again in agreement with the Canadian team.

Red Meat & Other Cancers

The greatest, undisputed risk factor for lung cancer is smoking, and other airborne pollutants are likely to be strongly associated too. In 2009 a research group[327] also established a link between red meat intake and lung cancer risk. This link was independent of whether it was red or processed meat that was consumed. It was also found that the risk was strongly associated with intakes of the substances formed in cooked meats, such as heterocyclic amines. It was noted, however, that the association was not strong enough to be statistically significant in individuals who had never smoked (the investigators did not want smoking to be a confounding variable, and so they analysed this in addition to red meat intake).

Processed Meats

Whilst heterocyclic amines can be produced in all types of meats, and red meat contains a high concentration of heme-iron whether it is cooked or not, there are unique differences between fresh and processed meats which could be involved in risk for cancers. Nitrates are included as a preservative in meats, despite them being banned from other foods. They are even present in some otherwise 'organic' processed meats, including some organic brands of bacon and sausages. Nitrates are also produced within the body, and so questions have arisen regarding how much needs to be consumed before it is 'too much' and damage can result.

A recent study by a Norwegian group[82] compared a fresh meat diet with a vegetarian one, and a high-processed meat diet with a vegetarian one, and investigated the risks for colorectal cancer. Their assessment of risk was via analysis of faecal samples, which were tested for indicators of oxidative stress. The first interesting finding was that the vegetarian diets exhibited the greatest signs of damage to DNA, which was particularly noteworthy because vegetarians are more at risk of colorectal cancer than individuals who eat meat. This risk is associated with a very high intake of cruciferous vegetables, which in moderation are protective against various cancers, but contain some harmful substances that can damage the gut when taken in excess. The researchers concluded that although both fresh and processed meats increase the amount of nitrates produced within the body equally, processed meats increase the amount of oxidative damage to DNA[82].

A study by a French group[83] published in 2010, reported that meats cured using nitrates increased the risk of carcinogenesis in the colons of rats, which is in agreement with the studies mentioned here, and supports the hypothesis that it is the nitrates specifically which increase risk of colorectal cancer. Substances related to nitric oxide, known as nitroso compounds, have also been hypothesised to increase cancer risk. These compounds can be formed within the intestines following consumption of red meat[84].

Iron, Oxidative Stress & Cancer Risk

Another potential route for increased cancer risk from red meat relates to its content of heme-iron. Excess iron is not easily removed from the body during normal processes (it can be lost through bleeding), and increased levels of iron could increase the generation of free radicals, which would increase oxidative stress and thereby increase risk of cancer development (along with various other negative consequences, such as reduced cardiovascular health, diabetes and inflammatory disorders such as arthritis).

Although this potential link is often referred to in the literature, there is very limited supporting evidence[69]. A recent study that did investigate this[85] did not find an association between increased red meat and heme-iron intake and markers of oxidative stress. In fact, the researchers reported that oxidative stress actually decreased when some carbohydrates were replaced by lean red meat. Further, the findings of that study did not support the idea that red meat and heme-iron intake promote inflammation. Part of the reason suggested for this is that for iron to cause damage it has to be circulating freely in the blood, but the body has developed effective mechanisms to have substances bind onto iron, ensuring the risk of damage from free iron is minimised.

Red Meats Compared with White Meats

In a study by an Australian group[80], rats were fed diets high in red meat, white meat, or starch. Both cooked red and white meats were found to induce DNA damage, with the amount of damage increasing with the amount of meat consumed, but the white meat caused significantly less damage than the red meat. The researchers noted that fibre was protective against this damage, and that although the rat's digestion does not perfectly represent that of humans, the findings are at least of relevance, supporting the idea that further research in human subjects is required. A study of red meat and poultry intake in human subjects[79], reported that the amount of poultry consumed was not associated with colorectal cancer risk, and noted that this was regardless of how well-done the meat was.

One Final Study

In 2009, a research group in America[81] published a paper based on over half-a-million subjects, all aged between 50 and 71 at the start of the study, and who were monitored at the beginning and end of a ten-year period. During that time, amongst their half-a-million subjects there were 47,976 male deaths and 23,276 female deaths. It was found that individuals with the highest intakes of red meat were likely to eat a higher amount of processed meat and a lower amount of white meat, have a higher intake of total calories, total fat and saturated fat, be a smoker, be overweight or obese, consume fewer fruits, vegetables and fibre, and have a lower level of education.

After correcting for those variables, red meat and processed meat were independently associated with an increased risk of mortality, including death from cancer and cardiovascular disease. White meat intake tended to be protective against total death, cancer deaths and all other causes of mortality. A small increase in risk for cardiovascular disease was noted for men with a higher intake of white meat.

* * * * * * *

Although there are sometimes conflicting findings when individual cancer types are analysed, that red meat intake is associated with an overall risk of cancer is fully supported by the scientific literature. In order for tumours to develop it is necessary for there to be repeated exposures to whatever it is that promotes their development[70].

Overall, it seems fairest to conclude red meat should be consumed no more than twice a week; it should not be overcooked, and should preferably come from pasture-fed animals. The remainder of the diet should comprise oily fish, organ meats, poultry, and fresh fruit and vegetables. With organ meats, poultry and fish there are no such upper limits that have been identified, although it can be maintained that no foods should be overcooked or charred, and all animal products should ideally come from animals not exposed to growth promoters.

The mechanisms responsible for increasing cancer risk from meats appear to be linked to heterocyclic amines and nitroso compounds. Specifically, it is the heating of food that generates these carcinogens, and their production can be exacerbated following interactions within the stomach. Because cooking meat is a fairly recent habit – in the perspective of several millions of years of consuming raw meat – we have not yet developed effective defences against the carcinogens formed. On balance, it would appear healthiest to limit red meat intake to no more than twice a week, and to cook the food with low-to-moderate heat and over as short a period of time as possible.

Fats

***"American consumers have no problem with carcinogens,
but they will not purchase any product, including floor wax,
that has fat in it."***

- Dave Barry

Fats are essential for health. They are structural components of the walls of every cell in the body, maintain the health of the blood vessels, are used to make hormones and other chemical messengers, transport fat-soluble vitamins (A, D E and K) and are required for healthy nerves and proper healing and control of inflammation. Most importantly, our brains require fats for the health of the cells, and certain types have been associated with improved behaviour and learning, whereas deficiencies have been associated with memory and learning deficits, and increased risk of depression and age-related degenerative conditions, such as arthritis, Parkinson's and Alzheimer's disease, and cognitive decline[328,329]

Fats are made up of fatty acids, and these can be classified according to their structure, so we have saturated and unsaturated types. The unsaturated fats can be sub-divided into mono-unsaturated and poly-unsaturated, and these terms all refer to the number of carbon bonds within the fatty acid's structure. Fats are mostly made of hydrogen and carbon, with bonds linking them together. There are single bonds throughout a saturated fat, and one (mono) or more (poly) double-bonds linking carbons in unsaturated fats[*].

---

[*] Take a look on Google Images for 'saturated unsaturated double bond' for examples of these fats

The unsaturated fats can be further subdivided according to whether they belong to the omega-3, omega-6 or omega-9 series fatty acids. These again are structural classifications, and are themselves composed of different fatty acids. Oleic acid is the omega-9 fatty acid found in olive oil, and is mono-unsaturated. The omega-3 and omega-6 fats are both poly-unsaturated, and because they cannot be manufactured within the body – yet are essential for health – they are deemed to be *essential* fatty acids. That is, we need to obtain sufficient amounts of both in our diets in order to be fully healthy.

Omega-3 and omega-6 series fatty acids play important roles in the health of our brain and nervous system, our skin and hair, bone health, healing and inflammation, metabolism and reproduction. Both these types of poly-unsaturated fats are required for complete physical and mental health

In general, unsaturated fats are considered to be healthier than saturated fats. The latter are found mostly in farmed meats, dairy, eggs and some plant oils (including palm oil and coconut oil). Unsaturated fats are found mostly in fish and vegetable oils. However, in nature all of these fats can be found in different foods, with differences really being in which sorts of foods have the most of whichever type. Further, the idea that it is the type of fat which is harmful is really over-simplifying the issue, because what it comes down to is that some foods are healthier than others, and what we actually eat can be healthy or not depending on the level and type of processing.

Modern agricultural techniques have led to the manipulation of meat away from its most natural state, although recently the agricultural scientists have done much to generate a swing back in the direction of more natural and beneficial fat compositions of meats. Still though, farmed meats contain an unnaturally high level of total fat compared to that of wild animals. Other common sources of fats include fish, dairy products, eggs, vegetable oils, nuts and seeds.

The omega-3 and omega-6 series fatty acids would have been obtained mostly from the brains, bone marrow and other organ meats of animals. Populations living in coastal regions would likely have obtained a great deal of their essential fats from fish. In fact, due to the direction modern societies have taken, it is very unusual to find animal brain and bone marrow easily available, and it no doubt creates an emotional response along the lines of revulsion, which has nothing to do with what it is like to actually eat these foods and everything to do with our perception of eating it. Nowadays most people obtain their omega-3 fats from fresh, oily fish, and this is certainly the easiest recommendation. There are of course problems with having too much fish, but all will be discussed in good time.

The omega-3 fatty acids do exist in nuts and seeds, but these foods are not ideal sources. Part of the problem relates to the specific types of omega-3 and omega-6 fats. Unlike proteins, which are managed and controlled via genetic factors, it is predominantly dietary factors which control the levels and functions of fats within our cells. These poly-unsaturated fats compete with each other for use within cells, which leads to different reactions taking place according to which fat is most available. Healing, for example, is most efficient if it is via the omega-3 system rather than the omega-6 system, although both are essential for total body health. This has facilitated the idea that there must be an ideal ratio of omega-3 to omega-6 fats, with people in westernised cultures consuming a ratio far higher in omega-6s to omega-3s than the roughly equal ratio we evolved with (up to 20 to 1 versus an evolutionarily more natural 1 to 1)[330,331].

This matter has since been further complicated, because there are different types of omega-3 and omega-6 fats, and current research is exploring how these interact with each other, meaning that rather than focussing on the overall ratio of omega-3s to omega-6s, there are sub-ratios within both which have to be managed. The types of which we need to increase or decrease our intake of will depend upon our health and lifestyle – if we are an athlete we might want the fats in different ratios to someone who is sedentary and suffering from arthritis, or someone suffering with depression or cognitive developmental deficits. This is an area where more research is required, but that research has to be of high enough quality for the findings to be truly meaningful. A recent review paper[86] has addressed many of the inconsistencies and misconceptions with research into the omega-3 fats[*].

One concern with nuts and seeds is that they tend to be very low in omega-3 fats and very high in omega-6 fats. However, the actual amounts that become active within the body are incredibly low. So, even though there is a high omega-6 fat content, these are not readily synthesised in the body into active forms, meaning the usefulness of those fats is very low. The fats in fish, by contrast, are readily synthesised into active forms, hence they are such a good source of their omega-3 fatty acids.

Nuts and seeds featured to such a minimal extent during our own evolutionary pasts that we never developed a digestive physiology efficient at breaking them down and utilising the fats. Hence, even omega-3 oils in supplement form lead to incredibly low levels of activity within the body if derived from seeds (such as flaxseed), as opposed to fish oils.

Vegetable oils are better-absorbed fats, but, similar to nuts and seeds, are typically much higher in omega-6s than omega-3s. Further, the processing of vegetable oils, which typically involves the use of heat, damages the oils and can make them harmful to us[87]. The

---

[*] Dr Simon Dyall – an academic and researcher in this field – is planning to write a book specifically on omega-3 fatty acids, although a publication date has not yet been confirmed

worst culprits are the vegetable fats used in the preparation of foods in some restaurants, particularly where foods are deep-fat fried. Having already been heated up during the initial processing, the fats are then heated at high temperatures and in some cases for hours within the facility, perhaps re-used over a few days, after which they might be taken away to be filtered and re-used. If oils have been heated and damaged, whether or not that damage will lead to harm to us once ingested will be dependent upon the type of fat[88].

Olive oil is regarded as healthy because it is low in the sorts of oils we should want to limit our intake of, and has been shown to have anti-carcinogenic properties[89]. Olive oil contains a high concentration of omega-9 fatty acids, appears to be more stable than most other oils, and generates fewer carcinogens when heated. Olive oil should be extra virgin, as this will have been prepared without being heated, and is best used as a dressing rather than as a cooking oil. However, if oil does have to be used then a small amount of either extra virgin olive oil or coconut oil[*], cooked at a low temperature for the shortest amount of time, would be favourable to other oils. Butters are even more stable, and may therefore be the preferred fat with which to cook. However, as the healthier options for cooking foods do not require the use of any fats, this issue becomes no more than a moot point.

* * * * * * *

In summary, fats are essential for the structure of our cells, our hormones and our overall health, particularly the omega-3 and omega-

---

[*] Coconut oil is also more stable than many other oils, and is understood to be less carcinogenic following heating

6 series fatty acids. Omega-3 fats have been shown to be protective against depression, behavioural problems, and the age-related decline in cognitive health, and may be protective against Parkinson's disease and Alzheimer's disease[90]. They are important for nourishing the brain and supporting learning and proper development. The total and saturated fat composition of farmed meats is higher than wild alternatives, although developments in farming are focussed on improving the fat content of meats. The most beneficial fats can be found in the bone marrow and brain of animals, although it is probably most appropriate to recommend people obtain their essential fats from small fresh oily fish. Because of the importance of omega-3 fatty acids, for those unable to obtain these from fish it is preferable instead to take them as fish oil supplements.

Fish

"I think fish is nice, but then I think rain is wet,
so who am I to judge?"

-Douglas Adams

Fish have been receiving a bad press over the years, based mostly upon evidence of pollutants in the sea being present in them, which subsequently get absorbed through the human gut and into the blood. Farmed fish have also received some negative attentions, most recently following the awareness campaign of Hugh Fearnley-Whittingstall and his 'Fish Fight'. Although the main thrust of his television series on the subject was the amount of caught fish being wastefully discarded (which has since caused the European Union to rethink this practice), coverage was also given to farmed fish.

The antibiotics given to fish present us with similar concerns to those from growth promoters used in animal farming. The colour of farmed salmon is augmented by colourants in their food pellets, and those colourants then become a part of the flesh we eat. The greatest travesty of fish farming is that the fish pellets are made from smaller fish, the continual harvesting of which is endangering stocks that would not otherwise be at risk, and those smaller fish would be more beneficial to us than farmed salmon, on account of their much higher omega-3 oil content.

The consequence of fish farming seems to be that we are given fish lower in essential oils and which are likely to contain colourants and antibiotics, all at the expense of endangering stocks of the smaller, more oily fish that are more beneficial to us. As consumers, it is in our best interests to be more demanding when it comes to choice, rejecting farmed fish in favour of the more beneficial, cheaper small fish. Those small fish, as well as being higher in omega-3 fatty acids, also contain small bones, which are often unnoticeable once the fish has been cooked, and would most likely contribute the best source of calcium to our diets.

* * * * * * *

Not many people would consider a return to the ancient days of eating uncooked red meat, but over the last decade or so we seem to have discovered a taste for raw fish. There are two main concerns with eating raw fish: the first relates to the ingestion of any harmful substances that would otherwise be destroyed by cooking, and the second is the ingestion of nematode worm larvae. The second is the shortest topic, so will be dealt with first.

Nematodes live in the digestive tracts of marine mammals, from where their eggs are excreted, turn into larvae, and are then consumed by crustaceans. Fish then consume those crustaceans and the larvae migrate to the flesh, which can then be consumed by humans. The larvae can live within our digestive tracts, or else penetrate the stomach or gut and cause serious damage. The symptoms of infection include acute abdominal pain, nausea and vomiting, typically within hours of ingestion. If the larvae are not vomited free from the body and instead pass into the bowel, then more severe damage to the gut lining can result[91].

Nematode worms can be destroyed by freezing the fish at minus 20°C for five days, or minus 35°C for fifteen hours[91]. Normally, cooking would destroy nematode worms, but this is obviously not an option for those preferring to eat sushi. As regulations are in place to reduce the risk of worms from commercially available sushi, the risk is likely to be greater from sushi prepared from fresh ingredients at home. However, considering so much commercially available sushi is little more than white rice, pickled vegetables and acidic sauces, often with the most meagre sliver of fish, it is probably not a bad idea to make sushi at home, provided it has been kept in the freezer at below minus 20°C for at least five days beforehand. The added benefit of this is that the oils within the fish will not be damaged by freezing as they can be through cooking, but it is important to ensure the fish is as fresh as possible in any case. The oils become damaged even at room temperature, if left out for long enough (perhaps a day or so).

* * * * * * *

There has been an abundance of media attention regarding chemicals in fish. There are two broad types of chemicals we ought to be both aware of and concerned about: metals and plastics. The vast majority are environmental pollutants that have found their way into lakes, rivers and seas, and are ingested by small organisms, which are in turn ingested by larger fish, where the chemicals become a part of the fish's flesh. With canned fish, some metals can also be leeched from the cans into the fish during the sealing process, when the cans are exposed to extremes of temperatures, as well as over time, and following opening of the cans if the contents are not used straight away or removed to a non-metallic container.

Metals are tested for in both fresh and canned fish, and in many cases the metal content fits within safe upper limits.

Predictably, perhaps, this is not always so. The risk of these metals to human health will vary according to the type of metal, with some causing oxidative damage to blood vessels, cells and organs, including the kidneys, liver, brain and nerve cells. The health risks are greatest for pregnant women and children.

Canned bonito, sardines and mackerel produced in Turkey have been found to contain acceptable amounts of zinc, copper, tin, and iron, but some samples had lead, cadmium and iron above those limits[92]. Another study of Turkish canned fish by the same author[93] assessed the content of metals in anchovies and rainbow trout. It was found that for both fish species the content of zinc, copper, cadmium, tin and mercury were within safe limits*, but they exceeded the upper limits for iron and lead.

Canned salmon, sardines and tuna were tested in Saudi Arabia, with the finding that generally metal content increased according to fish size, with sardines having the lowest levels, then salmon, and tuna having the highest metal content[94]. For the foods tested in Saudi Arabia the metals checked were iron, cadmium, nickel, zinc, chromium, and iron, and all were within the permissible limits of the World Health Organisation (WHO).

A study that investigated the content of mercury in canned tuna in the United States[95], noted an increase in mercury content over time from 1998 to 2003, with a peak in 2001. Mackerel was found to contain significantly less mercury than tuna, which fits with the general trend that larger predatory fish contain a higher content of metals than smaller fish. It was also reported there were no significant differences between fish from cans packed with oil and those packed with water. The main finding was that the mercury content was above

---

* It is noteworthy that what constitutes a safe limit will vary from country to country, so there can be variation between studies when they describe what is or is not 'safe'

the FDA's (U.S. Food and Drug Administration's) upper limit, and so the authors concluded that systematic monitoring was required,

Generally, the consumption of fish during pregnancy confers a number of health benefits to the child, as assessed via a longer gestation period, increased birth weight and reduced risk of growth problems[96]. It has been clearly demonstrated that the intake of omega-3 fatty acids from fish is important for development of a healthy central nervous system and the prevention of behavioural disorders. However, an intake of fish containing high levels of metals – and mercury in particular – could be harmful to the developing foetus.

Mercury accumulates in fish and is absorbed very effectively across the human gastrointestinal tract (95% bioavailability)[96]. A fairly recent study[96] found a link between a high intake of mercury from fish and very premature delivery (less than 35 weeks). The greatest fish source of mercury was canned fish, both because of the type of fish consumed (i.e. salmon and tuna) and because of the quantities of canned fish consumed by comparison to fresh fish.

Other pollutants of concern include polychlorinated bisphenyls (PCBs) and related chemicals such as BADGE and BFDGE (bisphenol-A-diglycidyl ether and bisphenol-F-diglycidyl ether, respectively). The chemicals are found in plastics in the marine environment, the plastics themselves coming from discarded waste, including water bottles, plastic bags, and plastic fishing equipment. The presence of these chemicals has been reported in fish taken from the Adriatic[97] and European sources, including canned fish[98,99,100], with many of the chemicals above the safe upper limits. It was noted that in some cases the results showed an 'average' content of these substances that was very high, not because many of the samples were so contaminated, but because a few were so highly contaminated they skewed the average upwards.

All fish contain N-nitroso compounds that can be

carcinogenic and should preferably be limited in the diet. The actual content in fresh fish is very low, but levels increase during storage, and through the activity of certain enzymes and bacteria, although adding salts containing nitrates would be another route. Freezing fish increases the levels of a precursor to these compounds, but even though the levels increase dramatically their actual effect on the body is negligible[101].

In 2010, the British Food Standards Agency (FSA) put in place new regulations on the labelling of fish. The purpose of the regulations was to make it easier for consumers to see exactly what they were buying, whether it was farmed or caught from inland waters or out to sea, and, when it was caught at sea, from which sea. This is of particular benefit to individuals who prefer larger predatory fish, such as salmon or tuna, as it would be prudent to opt for wild rather than farmed sources, and preferably to vary the location where the fish was caught, so as to limit exposure to pollutants that happen to be particularly concentrated in one area compared to another.

* * * * * * *

So, there is a risk with fish consumption that we are exposing ourselves to various unwanted chemicals, but the benefits of a diet high in fish far outweigh the potential costs, particularly when that diet is focussed on the smaller fish, which contain more beneficial oils and less of the pollutants.

A diet high in oily fish has been shown to have all the benefits of red meat, whilst decreasing insulin levels, improving insulin sensitivity and improving cholesterol levels (specifically increasing the HDL-cholesterol levels)[102]. Another study[103] compared the effects of a fish versus red meat diet on iron levels, in iron-deficient women. This population is typically recommended to increase their red meat consumption to improve iron status, but the study showed no difference whether the women were on the high red meat diet or high fish diet. Importantly, more research is being produced which demonstrates links between low intakes of fish – and therefore a low intake of highly bioavailable omega-3 fats – and increased risk of age-associated cognitive decline[104] and Parkinson's disease[105].

Despite concerns over fish stored in cans, even some of these species have been shown to have a high content of the essential omega-3 fatty acids[106], namely saury, herring and sprat. The problem is that these oils may have been damaged during the heating processes involved in canning the fish. The total content of the oils is not as important as their quality, and that is poorly reported at present. It could be that relying on oily fish from cans is adequate provided the diet is high in fruits and vegetables, which would help protect against damage from heated oils. This is clearly a compromise to the more ideal fresh fish, but such a compromise is preferable to having no oily fish at all.

In conclusion, we should broaden our tastes to include a variety of fresh fish from various waters. Fresh fish is preferable over fish that has been canned or preserved. Although there has been considerable media coverage on the issues of metals and plastics in fish, on the whole the levels are within safe limits, and exposure can be further limited by preferring smaller, oily fish to larger predatory fish, such as tuna and salmon. Doing so will also promote a high intake of omega-3 fatty acids, and hopefully limit our reliance on farmed fish, which usually contain colourants and antibiotics.

The Fad, Fashion & Hype of Superfoods

*"The scientific truth may be put quite briefly; eat moderately,
having an ordinary mixed diet, and don't worry."*
- Robert Hutchison, 1932

Different foods can confer different benefits, whilst others might present particular challenges to the body. Hence, we have a requirement for variety and the avoidance of too much or too little of important foods. In the majority of examples, plant foods contain some nutrients of benefit, and some that in excess can be harmful. Overall, a combination of foods is important, not only for maximising intake of important nutrients and reducing total intake of harmful ones, but for overall pleasure and satisfaction in preparing and eating foods.

Our understanding of the benefits of foods has been fostered by both scientific and medical research. In conducting studies, it is difficult to determine where a particular effect (reduced risk of cancer, for example) comes from, as in real life people obviously consume diets containing various different foods, and it is difficult to determine if any one food is conferring all or the majority of benefits. So, attempts are made to better understand the underlying mechanisms (i.e., reduced oxidative stress), and then either supplement individuals with specific nutrients or else increase their intake of a food rich in that/those nutrients. One of the problems with supplementation, as discussed, is that beneficial effects of a single nutrient are rare, because in life benefits come from the *interactions* of many nutrients.

Cruciferous vegetables[*], in particular, have been reported to contain a rich source of nutrients protective against cancer. Although these vegetables, like others, are a good source of anti-cancer nutrients, such as carotenoids, fibres, vitamins and minerals, they are also a particularly rich source of glucosinolates, which are thought to be especially protective against cancers[13,42]. It might be worth adding that a high intake of cruciferous vegetables actually increases the risk of colorectal cancer, indicating that a moderate intake is better than either a high or low one (eating these a few times a week is better than eating them every day or less than just a couple of times a month).

Studies have reported that watercress might be protective against cancer[13,43], because watercress has been found to reduce damage to DNA and promote anti-oxidant status, by improving levels of carotenoids in the blood[43]. There is absolutely nothing wrong with this finding, and such studies are useful to our understanding of the beneficial effects of fruits and vegetables in protecting us against cancers.

The problem is that the media tends not to report that 'vegetables', or even 'cruciferous vegetables' increase anti-oxidant levels and are protective against cancers. The issue is that the media seems to adore hype, fads and fashions, and so reports that watercress *specifically* has these beneficial effects. Does this mean watercress is better than the other cruciferous vegetables, or other vegetables in general? Simply because it is the example of cruciferous vegetables the researchers decided to test does not mean they tested all the other vegetables beforehand and found it to be 'the best'. They wished to study the protective effects of cruciferous vegetables, and so chose one they could acquire in the amounts they needed, and which would

---

[*] Cruciferous vegetables include arugula, bok choy, broccoli, brussels sprouts, cabbage, chinese cabbage, collard greens, horseradish, kale, kohlrabi, mustard, radish, rutabaga, turnips, wasabi and watercress[13].

be agreeable to their subjects.

A recent study by an American team[44] found that another cruciferous vegetable, broccoli, was protective against bladder cancer, regardless of vegetable intake overall. In particular, it was found that raw broccoli was associated with the strongest effect. It might be thought that these effects were noted for the regular consumption of broccoli, but the study actually reported the strongest effects being between those who consumed broccoli at least once a month, compared with those who consumed it less than once a month[44]. Either the active ingredient(s) within broccoli are so potent they need only be included very occasionally, or else there were confounding variables the investigators did not consider.

Overall, the sort of fuzzy logic of the media tends to lend itself to *ad hoc* reports of a particular new superfood, when the reality is only ever that a general example of a food group – such as a cruciferous vegetable – happens to be beneficial. This reporting of superfoods (and, indeed, the associated supermarket labelling), is not an issue by itself, but if people are consuming too few fruits and vegetables already, then it would be a shame if they focussed on selection of only one or two types of vegetables, at the expense of all the others on offer. After all, the most important point is that the diet should be rich in many different fruits and vegetables, not just one or two.

Importantly, plants protect themselves to a degree by containing chemicals that could be harmful if consumed in high doses. This indicates that it is not just a matter of increasing total nutrient intake that is important, but limiting intakes of any one plant food that might increase concentrations of harmful substances. This should not seem unreasonable, when we consider that too much of anything tends not to be good for us.

Oxidative & Nitrosative Stress

"Rest is not idleness, and to lie sometimes on the grass
under trees on a summer's day, listening to the murmur of the
water, or watching the clouds float across the sky,
is by no means a waste of time."

- John Lubbock

The specialised functions of cells vary according to location and tissue type, but all have their own metabolic pathways for producing energy from foods or stored sources, and all have signalling pathways for sending messages within the cell. The metabolic processes lead to the generation of reactive oxygen species (ROS) and reactive nitrogen species (RNS); substances once thought to do only harm. These by-products of metabolism can become involved in the signalling pathways and reactions, affecting how the cell works. If too much ROS or RNS are produced this can lead to cell damage, either by interfering with signalling pathways in a negative way, or directly by harming DNA, proteins, fats and other structures within the cell, including the cell's protective wall.

Oxidative and nitrosative stresses are associated with the production of reactive substances and free radicals[238]. Free radicals become involved in subsequent reactions, in which more reactive substances are formed. For those with an interest in chemistry, it might be appropriate to concede that although *oxidative* stress is the generally accepted term, oxidation reactions do not occur without reduction reactions, meaning that, as has been pointed out by various researchers, really the issue is oxidative *and* redox stress[238,239,240,241,242]. Nitrogen contributes to stress in a similar manner, and for the sake of clarity I will maintain use of 'oxidative stress' and 'nitrosative stress' to ensure completeness. I hope the chemists will appreciate my reasons for this and forgive my simplicity.

Historically, it was thought that ROS and RNS performed only negative functions within the body[238]. However, despite the bad press – some of which has been well deserved – the reality is that life is more complicated. Both ROS and RNS play important roles in cell signalling[238,243], and behave according to signals they receive within a cell. For example, nitric oxide can be an RNS that causes DNA damage, but it is also protective and happens to be critical for the health and function of blood vessels and various other tissues, including those of the nervous system. Free radicals are irreplaceable in their role in certain immune functions, including phagocytosis, where potentially harmful bacteria are ingested into immune cells that digest them[238]. A small amount of ROS and RNS is needed for optimal health of cells, and therefore the body as a whole[240].

Reactive oxygen and nitrogen species are important for the normal, healthy functioning of the respiratory, immune, neurological and reproductive systems[238,243]. Under normal circumstances, if any *excess* ROS or RNS are produced, they are neutralised by anti-oxidant defence enzymes, which scavenge them and prevent damage from occurring[243]. So, some substances can be anti-oxidants, meaning they oppose oxidative or nitrosative damage to cells, whereas others can be pro-oxidant, if they promote oxidative and nitrosative damage. Further, some ROS and RNS can be either anti-oxidative or pro-oxidative, depending upon requirements and signalling within a particular cell.

Oxidative and nitrosative stress result when there is an imbalance between generation of ROS and RNS, and the anti-oxidant scavengers that are expected to neutralise them. It appears the problem results more from increased generation of ROS and RNS, rather than reduced inactivation of them by scavengers[243].

Attempts to limit oxidative and nitrosative damage using supplementation have met with limited success, and in some cases even produced more harm than good[244]. It is more effective to reduce the generation of ROS and RNS, rather than try to deal with them once they are already in excess. This is particularly so as some ROS and RNS are essential for the maintenance of healthy cells, and trying to reduce them could interfere with normal physiologic functions and result in more damage[245,243]. Even high levels of vitamin C (ascorbic acid) have been suggested to have pro-oxidant effects, by interfering with the balance of normal oxidative processes[246]. This finding suggests that not only do ROS and RNS have double functions, but so too do anti-oxidants, which can become pro-oxidants under certain conditions[238].

How this can best be managed will depend upon which cells are generating too much oxidative and nitrosative stress, but, as a general approach, increased aerobic physical activity can reduce stress from ROS and RNS on the cardiovascular and respiratory systems, and support immune function. Too much exercise, beyond a level from which the body can efficiently recover from, can cause more harm (although few, if any, elite athletes would claim they are truly at their healthiest just before an important competition, when the balance of their training is tipped in favour of volume over recovery).

During normal physical activity, ROS and RNS are involved in anti-oxidant signalling, muscle excitation and muscle contraction. Oxidative and nitrosative stress is therefore essential for the health and proper functioning of muscles, and is involved in promoting anti-oxidant activity to prevent harm. This is not the case, however, when exercise is so stressful as to generate high levels of stress within muscle cells[238], such as high-intensity aerobic or resistance exercise.

Because exercise leads to favourable adaptations that limit oxidative and nitrosative stress, it is probably more appropriate to focus on gradually increasing intensity of physical activity over time, and promoting health and recovery by including plenty of proteins, essential fats, fruits and vegetables in the diet. This would certainly be preferable to taking high doses of anti-oxidant supplements, which could potentially interfere with normal anti-oxidant signalling and cause more harm[246,238]. Omega-3 supplementation has been shown to have no significant effects on oxidative stress or inflammation during exercise in trained men, although omega-3s can reduce resting signs of inflammation[240]. The authors of that study[240], suggested this finding was due to an already improved anti-oxidant and anti-inflammatory capacity of these men, who were used to training and so well-adapted and prepared for the stresses of exercise.

Consuming alcohol, smoking and air pollutants can increase oxidative and nitrosative damage, whereas fruits and vegetables are protective. A recent study from Indian researchers[247] found that zinc oxide was responsible for an increase in ROS within liver cells, and this was associated with an increase in cellular DNA damage[247]. Some chemicals found in cosmetics and other commonly used products can also increase stress from ROS and RNS. Zinc oxide is used in many consumer products, including cosmetics, sunscreens, skin creams, and aerosols. A quick Google search suggests it is even recommended by a website for homemade, natural herbal products, as an effective alternative to normal deodorants. Chronic liver injury and inflammation have been associated with an increased risk of liver cancer, although the mechanisms underlying this are poorly understood[248]. It would seem logical to want to avoid substances such as zinc oxide that increase oxidative stress in the liver.

Importantly, fruits, vegetables and omega-3 fatty acids all

support immune and nerve function, and promote recovery from injury, inflammation and physical stress, whereas some foods and diet strategies promote the production of ROS and RNS. A recent study [240] showed that a high intake of sugar (150 grams of dextrose) or a moderate amount of fat (33 grams) did not increase oxidative stress in the blood of healthy men, whereas a higher fat intake (66 grams) did increase oxidative stress. The study only assessed oxidative stress in the blood, and not other areas that might have been affected (such as blood vessel walls, cholesterol or the liver). So we know that excessive exercise is harmful, as are some substances commonly found in cosmetics and other products, and a high fat intake can also increase oxidative stress, although the extent of this is not yet fully understood.

* * * * * * *

Ketone bodies are an alternative source of energy to glucose, and the main fuel for the brain during the suckling period. The brain becomes more dependent upon glucose and less upon ketones as it matures[249]. When some normal systems fail, such as the ability to use glucose for energy, or when adopting a ketogenic diet*, the use of ketones for energy increases.

Ketone bodies have been shown to have the capacity to scavenge excess ROS, which might be how ketogenic diets can protect nerve cells from damage and be beneficial for individuals with certain conditions, such as epilepsy and some neurodegenerative diseases[249].

This is a useful and important finding, as it demonstrates that

---

* A low carbohydrate diet that promotes the formation of ketones for energy

individuals unable to benefit from the anti-oxidants found in fruits and vegetables still have the capacity to protect themselves from oxidative stress. Whilst this is a benefit to individuals who suffer from particular conditions, it is still more beneficial for most people to have a normal diet, containing plenty of fruits and vegetables, which have a high protective capacity and confer the additional benefits of providing important dietary fibres. Further, a recent study by British and American investigators[250] reported a mechanism by which ketones can actually fuel the growth of tumours and promote cancer development. In fact, the benefits of ROS protection from ketone bodies are likely to be far out-weighed by potential problems, and this finding comes from the results of investigations into fasting-based 'therapeutic' diets.

Fasting and severe caloric restriction feature as the basis of some diets. During these conditions there is an insufficient supply of carbohydrates to meet energy requirements, necessitating the body to utilise alternative sources of energy. In response to fasting the body releases fats stored in the liver, muscles and fat cells. Fats released into the blood are converted in the liver into ketones, which become the essential source of energy for the muscles, brain and other tissues.

Ketone bodies are acidic, and their release into the blood would typically trigger a feedback loop to limit and control their production. However, in type 1 diabetics and during fasting this process is inadequate because the body continues to require energy. So, fasting leads to increased ketone production, which has the potential to increase the acidity of the blood (ketoacidosis), placing increased demands on the kidneys and bone minerals to maintain a normal blood pH.

The increased fats in the liver increase the risk of hepatic steatosis (fatty liver disease), once considered to be benign but since associated with symptoms similar to those observed in alcohol-

112

induced liver disease. Even short-term fasting (24-72 hours) increases fats in the liver, which has been associated with inflammation and fibrosis, following increased ROS and RNS production[251,252].

A variety of markers of oxidative stress have been found to be elevated following short-term fasting. These have been implicated with acute liver damage, due to increased ROS produced by the cells' mitochondria in response to the altered energy-producing pathways. Further, there is not only an increase in production of ROS and RNS, but the ability for our natural scavengers to neutralise these is reduced.

That short-term fasting increases the rate of ROS and RNS production is a serious consequence, but that our inherent ability to protect ourselves is significantly reduced makes the scope of the problem far worse. The liver is efficient at regenerating itself after damage, but the acute liver injury and increased fibrosis is a problem beyond this, as these events are consequences of damage beyond what the liver can effectively control. So, we have mitochondria within the liver cells producing more free radicals (ROS and RNS) than normal, coinciding with a decreased ability to protect the cells from damage[253] and an increased release of pro-inflammatory chemicals[252].

The scope of damage is further increased because proteins are utilised for energy as well, and again it has been shown that in the fasting condition the proteins become damaged, and there is then interference with normal cell signalling processes and the natural RNS scavengers are altered, rendering them less active[251]. Worst of all, the sequence of events that increase oxidative and nitrosative damage generate self-increasing cycles, with the production of some leading to the production of more, and all the while with a decreasing ability for cell protection.

Although this all deals specifically with short-term fasting, low-blood glucose levels – as can be observed in type I diabetics – has also been associated with increased oxidative damage through similar pathways (in both cases low energy levels lead to increased fat release and the production of ketones in the liver)[254]. In fact, some of the negative effects are cumulative, in that women with diabetes have been found to suffer increased oxidative and nitrosative damage from fasting when compared to women without diabetes[255,256]. So, although there is some evidence of a protective effect of ketones, overall the benefits are small in number and magnitude when considered together with the harmful consequences. This supports the idea that ketogenic diets should only be recommended for those with specific disease conditions that alter the overall balance in favour of benefits with this type of diet. The evidence demonstrates that healthy individuals should not compromise their health by fasting or severely limiting their energy intake.

* * * * * * *

In addition to the benefits of fruits and vegetables, anti-oxidant capacity is also improved from other sources, including tea and coffee. In fact, tea and coffee contribute the greatest amounts of anti-oxidants in modern diets[*257]. It is unclear whether this is because people consume so much tea and coffee or so few fruits and vegetables. In any case, this demonstrates benefits of both teas and coffee, although the inclusion of milk into these will reduce the amount of anti-oxidants that can be absorbed into the blood.

Wine is also a contributor of anti-oxidants[257], and has been shown to be protective against conditions such as cardiovascular disease and some cancers. However, confounding variables can be an issue, as individuals who consume wine tend to have more money and

---

[*] Discussed further in the chapter on Teas and Coffee

a healthier diet in general than those with a lower income. On average, wine-drinkers consume more fruits and vegetables, and tend to have a healthier lifestyle than people who consume other types of alcohol. Even if all of the confounding variables are taken into account, alcohol itself (ethanol) may be protective, but alcohol is also a pro-oxidant and is harmful to the cells of the nervous system, brain and liver.

This implies that whilst there are some benefits to consuming alcohol, those benefits can also be derived from increasing intake of anti-oxidants from non-alcoholic sources, and in so doing avoiding the harm associated with alcohol consumption. In other words, alcohol can be included in the diet for many important reasons, but doing so entirely for its health benefits does not seem supported, particularly when considered from the perspective of whole body health.

Weight-loss in individuals who are obese has been found to reduce oxidative stress, improve obesity-related metabolic alterations in the liver, improve liver health, and improve omega-3 fatty acid activity and capacity[258]. Long-term oxidative stress in the livers of obese individuals has been related to increased fat within the liver, which can lead to more serious conditions and negatively affect liver function[241]. Diabetes mellitus has also been shown to be associated with increased oxidative stress in the liver[259], which could be responsible for decreased liver function[260]. Conversely, reducing oxidative and nitrosative stress should improve liver health.

* * * * * * *

Oxidative and nitrosative stress has been associated with cardiovascular disease, atherosclerosis, neurodegenerative diseases including Alzheimer's and Parkinson's, diabetes mellitus, metabolic syndrome, skin diseases, and psychic impairments such as schizophrenia and attention deficit hyperactivity disorder (ADHD). These stresses to our DNA and normal cell repair mechanisms are also involved in the ageing process[238].

Oxidative and nitrosative stress to the liver could be involved in increased overweightness and obesity, whereby the longer someone has been overweight the harder it becomes to lose weight, due to decreased effectiveness of organ systems following long-term oxidative and nitrosative stress. Some of the damage caused by ROS and RNS may be initiated by gene mutations in the mitochondria, leading to overproduction of ROS and RNS, which could in turn cause further damage to the mitochondria and the rest of the cell[239]. The mitochondrial DNA of skin cells can be damaged by oxidative stress caused by sunlight, and this has been related to ageing of the skin and cancer development[261].

In the short-term, oxidative and nitrosative stress is not of serious concern, because the repair mechanisms can be effective during recovery periods. However, long-term stress can increase the likelihood that protective, inhibitory and repair systems will be overwhelmed, permitting damage to proteins, fats, and DNA, ultimately leading to damage to cells, organs and organ systems. This could result in chronic inflammation and the onset and development of the serious diseases mentioned in this chapter[238].

Oxidative and nitrosative stress might also be involved in adverse reactions to anaesthetics, and preventing this may help prevent anaesthetic-induced brain cell death[262]. Protecting against oxidative and nitrosative stress has been shown to protect brain cells of developing animals from damage[262]. However, brain cells should adapt to normal stresses in any case, so as to increase protection against such damage[263].

Various maternal infections have been implicated in premature delivery, which in itself is associated with poor health of the infant and increased risk of serious disorders. Antibiotics are frequently administered to treat the infections, but these carry risks to the baby, including cerebral palsy[263]. There is growing evidence that a consistently high level of oxidative stress in the mother might contribute to premature delivery and foetal death[263].

There is growing evidence that increased oxidative stress interferes with signalling pathways within blood vessels, preventing proper functioning of the vessel walls and ultimately contributing to cardiovascular disease[243]. More specifically, the anti-oxidant capacity of the blood vessels is decreased, and the generation of ROS, RNS and inflammation increases[242]. Atherosclerosis is associated with this response, whereby the blood vessels fail to function properly, normal signalling is disrupted, and the vessel walls lose their elasticity and promote local inflammation[242]. This cascade of events is also associated with oxidative stress to circulating cholesterol[264], which can adhere to the blood vessel wall and increase risk of thrombosis and clot formation.

Oxidative stress is a major factor in the onset of male infertility, with ROS damaging the forming sperm and harming both structural components of sperm and its DNA. Oxidative stress also harms certain cells of the testes, which are responsible for managing hormones important for the development of healthy sperm, thereby interfering with sperm development[265]. Oxidative stress might also be related to female infertility, but direct evidence is not currently available[266] and research is ongoing.

* * * * * * *

Although oxidative and nitrosative stress have negative effects on the body, it should be considered that this represents an imbalance rather than the way the chemicals themselves always behave. As has been discussed, a balance in favour of increased oxidative and nitrosative stress results in damage to wherever such stress occurs, such as within cells or blood vessels, and this can lead to systemic problems, such as reduced immune function, increased risk of cardiovascular disease, diabetes, arthritis and cancers. In pregnant women, an imbalance that results in increased oxidative stress can be responsible for infections, premature delivery and increased risk of severe health consequences in the foetus and newborn. These ill-effects all result from oxidative and nitrosative stress, specifically. The actual chemicals themselves that are involved, even those often classified as ROS and RNS, can have critical roles in protecting cells and blood vessels – and therefore us – from damage.

We have evolved various protective mechanisms against over-production of – and harm from – ROS and RNS. Naturally occurring substances within cells, which interfere with the enzymes generating ROS and RNS, normally prevent over-production. When these fail, there are other substances (generically termed anti-oxidants or free radical scavengers), which scavenge or trap excess ROS and RNS and render them harmless. If these protective systems are insufficient, the next step is removal or repair of whatever has been damaged[238].

In conclusion, ROS and RNS are essential, as are anti-oxidants and pro-oxidants. Anti-oxidants can behave as pro-oxidants, particularly (it seems) if high doses of single anti-oxidants are ingested, which can then interfere with normal cell signalling[238]. It is far more effective to prevent the excessive generation of ROS and RNS, rather than try to prevent their generation at all, or to ingest excessive amounts of anti-oxidant supplements, which could even have a pro-oxidant effect. The focus should be on ensuring the balance is in favour of preventing stress. This can be achieved by limiting exposure to high concentrations of harmful chemicals, increasing protective factors such as moderate aerobic physical activity and increased intake of fresh fruits, vegetables and omega-3 fatty acids, and reducing psychological stress.

"Good for the body is the work of the body, good for the soul the work of the soul, and good for either the work of the other."
- Henry David Thoreau

Human Milk

"A newborn baby has only three demands. They are warmth in the arms of its mother, food from her breasts, and security in the knowledge of her presence. Breastfeeding satisfies all three."
- Grantly Dick-Read

That human milk is the best possible nourishment for infants and young children is beyond question. In order to understand the virtues of any milk for human health, it is first necessary to describe this from its natural, most health-promoting perspective. Hence, appreciating the merits of human milk for infants becomes essential for understanding the place, if any, of dairy products for adults.

The human immune system is divided into two components: innate and acquired immunity. Broadly, the innate immune system is what we are born with, whereas acquired immunity relies upon interactions between the body and potentially harmful, or 'alien' substances, including food allergens, bacteria, fungi and viruses. Accumulating research shows there is a carry-over between innate and acquired systems, with the components of both being linked, making a true distinction not a real representation of how they work in life. However, it is sufficient to state that a foetus is protected from infection by the maternal immune system, and the newborn's immune system is deficient at birth and matures rapidly over the first months and years of life.

Since the 1970s, researchers have been aware that human milk contains active immune cells, and that breastfeeding permits the transfer of various immune factors from mother to infant[107]. These immune factors help protect the infant from colds, flu and common infectious diseases, including necrotising enterocolitis and Crohn's disease[107].

The ability for a mother to directly feed her newborns is a characteristic shared by all mammals. This is in difference to all other organisms, in which adults can supply food but the young have to be able to process those foods from birth, and have to have immune systems sufficiently developed to protect themselves from infections. The mammary glands themselves are highly specialised sweat glands, which have adapted over millions of years to be effective at secreting modified lactate.

Lactate is derived from carbohydrates, and many of us are familiar with it as the substance generated during high intensity physical activity, as a by-product of carbohydrate metabolism. What many people do not fully realise is that the liver is highly effective at recycling lactate back into glucose to help fuel further exercise. Sweating during exercise releases not only water for cooling, but many essential minerals too. That mammals have adapted to secrete lactate and essential minerals from highly specialised glands, over a period of more than a hundred million years, is not as improbable as it might otherwise appear. Also from an evolutionary perspective, milk that confers the most benefits to the newborn can be expected to increase the survival chances of the infant, and so over time evolutionary pressures have led to human milk being highly specific for the health of newborns.

Milk is a rich source of carbohydrates, fats, proteins and essential micronutrients. The presence of immune factors specific to the development of the human immune system is something fairly well understood, which has led to recommendations of minimum time periods before weaning, to promote transfer of minimal levels of acquired immune factors from mother to child.

* * * * * * *

Much of the research since the 1970s has supported the association between breastfeeding and protection of infants against infections, particularly infections of the gastrointestinal and respiratory systems[108]. More recently, it has been found that this goes beyond the simple transfer of active immune cells.

It appears that various substances are transferred to the infant, which actively promote the overall development of the child's immune system[108], including anti-inflammatory components[109,110,111]. Most importantly, these substances survive the infant's digestive processes, and lead to functional effects in the body[109]. In addition to active immune cells, there are also growth factors, hormones and other chemical messengers, and the list of identified immune-system-specific substances in milk is growing rapidly[108,111].

The carbohydrates in human milk have been found to be important for the health of the infant's developing gut, and influence the acquisition and growth of the gut's microfloral ecosystem[110]. Because cows' milk either does not contain these particular carbohydrates, or else contains them in such low levels that they cannot be detected, the guts of infants receiving cows' milk will not be protected as effectively as infants raised on breastmilk[110].

The proteins in milk are essential for promoting the growth of the infant's muscles, bones and connective tissues. They also carry out various other physiological functions, promote the development of a healthy gut, enhance the immune system, and protect against potentially harmful bacteria, yeasts and viruses[112]. Some of these proteins have also been reported to protect against tumours[112].

Bacteria are essential for human health. Their ecosystem within the digestive tract does not only support them but promotes our own health too. Many infections, diseases and disorders can follow from imbalances in this system, with bacteria responding to the health of their 'host' and the host responding to the health of the bacteria. There are approximately 100 trillion bacterial cells in the average human, compared with 10 trillion human cells. This does not include the mitochondria within each of our cells, which behave as a bacterial component in their own right, having their own DNA, reproducing independently of the cell, and supplying our cells with energy without which we could not survive.

The health of the adult human gut is founded, facilitated and developed from early infancy, and carbohydrates, proteins and various immune factors transfer from breastmilk to promote this development. Importantly, it is not simply the physical framework that is developed, but the type of bacteria that predominate in the infant's gut will also be influenced by his or her exposure to breastmilk. The recent increases in the incidence of allergic, autoimmune and other immune function-related diseases demonstrates the need to support the bacteria already residing within the gut, thus signifying the importance of breastfeeding for infants[113].

Interestingly, in infants, a high intake of the minerals calcium and phosphorous can be harmful, because they contribute to an acidic environment that the developing kidneys cannot effectively correct. As a result, human breastmilk is very low in phosphorous content compared with the milk of other mammals, and it is thought that a low content but high intestinal absorption are important for infant health[114]. A disturbance in this balance could lead to the presence of harmful bacteria in the gut, an acidic environment in the blood, potentially harmful effects on blood vessels and bones, and an increased risk of infections[114].

* * * * * * *

The growth of the infant formula market has distorted this message somewhat, with advertising common that implies 'follow-on' products are a natural part of the weaning process, and something that can apparently happen early on. We have been something of a victim of media and societal pressures in this regard, because it is the norm in free-living, non-westernised populations around the world for mothers to breastfeed their children until they are around three or four years of age, coinciding with a very gradual and progressive weaning onto whole foods. Only women unable to breastfeed really 'require' alternatives to human milk for their children, and whilst this is a group who require sound, evidence-based information regarding what is most appropriate, the message that infant formulas and other 'baby foods' are normal for all infants is a nonsense. Although there is unfortunately no scope to develop this issue further within this book, it should be made clear that some mothers will have a requirement to use alternatives to breastmilk. Unfortunately, at present there is a lack of research to aid informed decision-making on this issue.

In reality, infants should be raised on breastmilk until they are ready to be weaned onto whole foods, processed at home from fresh ingredients. Although there can be exceptions to this, the message people in westernised societies receive seems to be based on pressure from manufacturers and media, which ultimately encourages changes that later affect peer pressure, as opposed to a reflection of what is in the best interest of the family as a whole, and the developing child in particular.

Current recommendations should be based upon our

understanding of the health requirements of the newborn, and will doubtless be adjusted as we learn more about the health benefits that come later in life from breastfed infants and young children[111]. Human breastmilk is the gold standard which formula foods aim to replicate. Considering how our knowledge of breastmilk composition is being continually improved, it will be a long time indeed before infant formulas can in any way compare with breastmilk, and even then it can only be in terms of the simple nutrients – it will be far harder to create a formula containing the complex organic messengers, particularly as a mother's milk will vary in composition according to specific factors for her own child[115]. At present, infant formulas have been found to contain far more calories than breast milk[117], suggesting that they miss the target at even the most basic level.

A recent comparison of mothers of girls and boys[115], found that mothers produce milk containing 25% more energy for sons compared to daughters. This could account for the higher initial growth rates that have been observed for boys compared to girls[115]. Milk from mothers who gave birth to premature infants has been shown to be 20-30% higher in total energy and fat content, 15-20% higher in proteins, and approximately 10% lower in lactose[116]. These findings suggest that the production of milk and its composition is highly variable, and alters according to the requirements of the infant.

"If a multinational company developed a product that was a nutritionally balanced and delicious food, a wonder drug that both prevented and treated disease, cost almost nothing to produce and could be delivered in quantities controlled by the consumers' needs, the very announcement of their find would send their shares rocketing to the top of the stock market. The scientists who developed the product would win prizes and the wealth and influence of everyone involved would increase dramatically. Women have been producing such a miraculous substance, breastmilk, since the beginning of human existence."

- Gabrielle Palmer

Dairy

"Cheese is milk's leap towards immortality."

- Clifton Fadiman

Despite dairy being a common component of many modern diets, animals have only been farmed for a few thousand years – a mere blink of the eye in terms of human evolution – and the routine consumption of dairy products has an even more recent history. This is evident in that the majority of people in the world are unable to digest lactate after childhood[118].

Recommendations to maintain dairy intake throughout life stem from the idea that dairy is important for bone health[119]. Although bone health itself is the subject of the next chapter, it is impossible to deal with dairy without discussing bone health too. For this reason there will be some carry-over between these two chapters, but this has been considered to be better than leaving important points undeveloped.

Following childhood, a healthier spectrum of proteins, essential oils and carbohydrates should preferably come from fresh meats, fish, fruits and vegetables. Human milk has evolved to be very effective at nourishing newborns into young children, but lacks the macronutrients required by older children. It also lacks the rich spectrum of phytonutrients that come from fruits and vegetables. It should therefore be no surprise that dairy products are even further from the mark.

The human brain is highly dependent upon essential fatty acids, and the requirements of calves do not compare in this regard.

Further, because humans generally lack the ability to effectively digest milk following early childhood, the bioavailability of some of the nutrients in milk decreases, and the absorption of nutrients from other foods can be reduced if consumed with milk. In reality, the only reason people are recommended dairy products following early childhood is on the understanding that it is healthy, but the only perceived health benefit is for bone health, and that is entirely based upon milk's calcium content.

Up until early childhood, infants and young children would benefit far more from human breastmilk, which has evolved over millions of years to be the best available substance for supporting growth and development. The complexities of the human gut, immune system and brain make any milk other than human breastmilk either less healthy or even harmful to the young. Exposure of infants to proteins founds in cows' milk has been shown to generate unusual immune responses in the developing child, which increase the risk of developing type 1 diabetes[120].

To conclude this introduction, humans have had limited exposure to dairy products in an evolutionary sense, and just as human breastmilk has evolved to be the best available substance for developing human infants into children and subsequently healthy adults, so cows' milk has evolved to be the best substance for the guts, immune systems and brains of calves growing into cows. The pasteurisation process does not destroy all of the immune and growth factors, leaving some hormones and bacteria active, and meaning that when humans consume this we are exposing ourselves to some very unusual chemicals and bacteria, which can then have an effect on our own gut health, immune systems, and development.

The only conceivable reason for humans to consume cows' milk is if infants need a breastmilk substitute, in which case we must favour the product that has been processed to the highest degree, to limit exposure to potentially harmful bacteria, hormones and other chemical messengers. That dairy is still recommended for bone health, however, is one of many issues requiring discussion. From an evolutionary perspective – for those who consider all milks to be equal and healthy for individuals of any age – bovine lactate is certainly not *natural* for adult humans. Considering dairy is being recommended against even for vegetarians[121], for whom this was once seen as an important source of proteins and minerals, there is clearly a requirement to review the evidence.

* * * * * * *

A fairly recent review article from American researchers[122], commented that dairy intake in the United States is amongst the highest in the world, comprising 72% of calcium intake. Despite this, the rates of osteoporosis and fractures are also very high. As a consequence, researchers and medical professionals are questioning the traditional idea that increasing calcium and/or dairy intakes can prevent osteoporosis and reduce fracture risk[122].

One of the suggested reasons that milk itself is not particularly useful for promoting bone health, is that its sodium content competes with calcium uptake into the blood from the kidneys, ultimately leading to both being eliminated from the body in the urine. In agreement with other studies mentioned in this chapter, the American review[122] reported that as long as people are consuming above the *minimum* levels of calcium required for bone health, there are no additional benefits of having more. Whilst a calcium intake below 400-mg a day has been found to be harmful to bone development, anything above 400-500-mg/day confers no additional benefits to bone mineral density or fracture risk in children or adolescents[122].

A study in New Zealand[123] reported that a high intake of dairy products significantly increased the bone mineral density and bone mineral content in the thighs and lower back of teenage girls. Following the end of the study period the girls returned to their previous levels of dairy consumption, below that which had increased their bone mineral density during the study, and demonstrated that enforced dieting practices are difficult to maintain in the long-term. This was an interesting finding, however, because another New Zealand group[124] reported that calcium supplementation from a dairy product had no significant effect on bone health, when the boys and girls tested already had a high intake of calcium anyway. This makes sense, because both genetic and environmental factors – rather than an excess of related dietary factors – determine bone mineral density.

So, genetics instruct bone cells to build bone, and they will build as much as the genetic code tells them to. How much of the actual building blocks are circulating in the blood is irrelevant, because the DNA blueprint is set to build bones of specific proportions, and just because someone has more calcium moving around, that is not a reason for the cells actively building the bones to build more.

By way of an example, if you were to have an architect with a blueprint for building a house, who lives within a room of his own nearby, he or she can only pass the blueprint over to the building contractors. There is no reason the architect or contractors should change the building just because someone over-ordered on the bricks. However, if there are not enough bricks to match the requirements of the plans, then there will be a problem. As far as the body is concerned, below the architect's minimum requirements for calcium there will be deficiencies in build quality, but calcium-deficiency does not really exist in modern societies because it is abundant in meats, fish and to a lesser degree in fruits and vegetables. That a study reported greater bone mass in teenagers consuming a high concentration of milk might indicate they were otherwise deficient in minerals, or else that as well as increasing their intake of dairy, they increased their amount of bone-building physical activity too. With the other study showing no effect of milk consumption, it is clear there is more to bone health than calcium intake alone.

The environmental factors are what really matter. Genetics cannot be affected from outside, but environmental stress, such as high-impact exercise, sends new chemical messages around the body, instructing muscles and bones to strengthen themselves beyond the basic genetic requirements. So, high-impact exercise can increase bone health, for which extra building blocks are required, but even then there are no benefits to be had from a high calcium intake, just as long as the new 'minimum' requirement is met.

* * * * * * *

Because of the bad press that dairy has been receiving some parents have sought alternatives to cows' milk. Again, the problem with cows' milk is that it has evolved to be highly specific for the development of calves into cows, and this is facilitated by a composition of more than just proteins, fats and carbohydrates. The hormones, other chemical messengers, immune factors and bacteria are all highly specific to the developing calf. Similarly, any alternative milk will be highly specific for the newborn it has evolved to nourish. In some cases it might not make any difference, but in others the effects could be disastrous. Goats' milk should no longer be available as an alternative for infants, because the effects (including severe allergic reactions) can be devastating[125]. Similarly, there are reports of young children admitted to hospital with terrible developmental problems (neurological disorders, reversal of normal growth and maturation, loss of motor skills and ability to walk), all resulting from parents giving them a diet high in obscure alternatives, such as rice drinks, vegetable infant foods, soy products and other vegan foods[126]. These problems are associated with nutrient and energy deficiencies, following on from exclusive intakes of these alternatives.

As has been already discussed, in an ideal world newborns should be fed breastmilk until early childhood, when they can be weaned onto natural whole foods. However, some parents do not live in an ideal world, and providing their children with everything they need to develop can sometimes involve compromises. Human breastmilk is the best possible source of nutrients for developing infants and children, and infant formulas aim to replicate this as much as possible, even though it is an impossible task, even with today's technology, to fully accomplish this.

Dairy products can cause problems, including an increased risk of developing type 1 diabetes in some children, and an increased risk of various gut and immune problems. It is difficult to say which is better (or least bad) for parents unable to breastfeed (or breastfeed enough), but there will be benefits and negative consequences of either infant formulas and cows' milk. Perhaps some of both? In any case, there is too much to discuss on this in a book concerning adult diets, so this has to be sufficient. Breast is best, and infant formulas and cows' milk present their own deficiencies and compromises. In any case, either of these latter two would be more appropriate than other alternative, non-human milk sources, and are safer and more appropriate than many milk-alternatives commercially available.

In older children and adolescents, there is no good quality evidence supporting a need or any real benefit of increased calcium or milk consumption for bone health[122]. Sufficient calcium for bone health can be derived from green leafy vegetables, fish and meats, from where it is absorbed at least as effectively as from cows' milk. Further, evidence does report an association between dairy intake and increased risks of diabetes, cancer, cardiovascular disease, stroke and acne during adulthood (to be discussed later in this chapter).

In terms of childhood fractures, a study by an Australian group [127] reported that milk was no better at preventing fractures in children than soft drinks, including cola. Importantly, any attempts to increase bone mass during childhood and adolescence will not generate lasting effects in later adulthood[128]. Children should have a good diet and spend as much time playing outside as can be managed, and this will support and promote bone health far more – and be far more beneficial for total health as well as disease prevention – than allowing them to be less active whilst providing them with calcium tablets or dairy.

Bone health is determined by genetic and environmental factors and, over time, bone mineral density will return to its genetically predetermined composition, in the absence of environmental stresses, such as physical activity. To reduce the risk of osteoporosis and fractures in later life, the most important recommendation is to be physically active in middle and older age, incorporating plenty of weight-bearing exercise and enjoying a good quality diet.

* * * * * * *

Cows' milk increases levels of the hormones insulin and insulin-like growth factor-1 (IGF-1) to a similar degree as high glycaemic index foods[129], which in itself increases risk of diabetes, inflammation and reduced cardiovascular health. Further, these hormones could have a negative effect on the glands that cause acne, and not only would a high milk intake thereby increase acne during adolescence, but could promote adult acne, which is associated with an increased risk of some cancers[129].

More recently, investigators[131] have reported on a link between milk intake of adult men and increased risk of prostate cancer, whilst others[132] have found no relationship between women's milk intake and breast cancer risk (interestingly, white cheese was found to be protective, although the authors did not speculate as to why this might have been). Interestingly, dairy intake has been associated with a decreased risk of colon cancer in adults[133] although there was no relationship to risk of rectal cancer. The underlying mechanisms of why this might have been were not discussed. It should not be unreasonable that there can be some benefits to dairy consumption, although more research is needed to support such a finding. Really it comes down to a balance between costs and benefits, and overall there appear to be more costs with dairy consumption compared to very few benefits.

A study of the bone health of post-menopausal women[134] noted that women with the lowest intake of milk were the most likely to smoke and consume alcohol. The authors also commented that this research was complicated by the fact that women with a family history of poor bone health were most likely to take supplements, meaning that whether supplements were effective or not in their own right was difficult to assess, because the analysis was of women who might be more susceptible to problems anyway.

What that study reported, though, was that women with the

highest intake of calcium had a slightly reduced risk of fracture compared to those with the lowest intake (more than 1200-mg/day compared to less than 600-mg/day)[134], but there was no relationship between milk consumption, specifically, and fracture risk. Calcium absorption from calcium supplements, milk, calcium-set tofu, sweet potatoes and beans were all about the same, but absorption was not as high from these as it was from green leafy vegetables[122].

The finding of a very high compared to very low intake having marginal benefits supports a comment already made, which is that as long as people are consuming the minimum calcium required, there are no additional benefits to consuming more. It was previously mentioned that an intake of calcium below 400-mg/day is likely to be insufficient, but there are no benefits to consuming any more than about 400-500-mg/day. In a study comparing an intake above 1200-mg/day to an intake below 600-mg/day, this lower level could have included people with intakes far below this minimum 400-mg/day threshold. It was just a shame they did not compare a group with an intake between 400- and 1200-mg/day.

Because calcium increases the risk of cardiovascular disease, stroke, diabetes and inflammatory problems, and milk independently increases the risk of some cancers, diabetes and cardiovascular disorders, it is difficult to claim a benefit of high dairy consumption. Further, a recent Swedish study[340] reported that the intake of whole milk and yoghurt increased the risk of stroke.

Increasing physical activity whilst maintaining a healthy diet is all that is required for promoting and maintaining optimal bone health. For those with a low calcium intake, it would be appropriate to increase consumption of green leafy vegetables, sweet potatoes, meats and fish, as these are not only a good source of highly bioavailable calcium, but are also rich in other important vitamins, minerals and other essential nutrients. Interestingly, the study comparing sub-600-mg/day of calcium to plus 1200-mg/day[134] reported a 33% reduced risk of fracture in post-menopausal women consuming dark fish (such as swordfish, mackerel, sardines, salmon and bluefish), more than once a week compared to those consuming them less than once a month.

Milk fortified with nutrients has been used to supplement the diet of elderly people at risk of nutrient deficiencies. A study by an Australian group[332] reported that six months of supplementation with milk fortified with extra calcium, folate and vitamin D had no effect on the bone health, muscle strength or mobility of elderly subjects. Although vitamin D levels did increase, this was not to a level thought useful to reduce risk of fractures. A recent meta-analysis[337] found no association between milk intake and risk of hip fractures. A similar finding was reported by an earlier meta-analysis[333], also reporting no relationship between milk intake and fracture risk. One of the findings of the study regarding adolescent girls and their milk intake[123], was that they did not maintain the higher intake after the study finished. This has also been noted in the elderly[135], suggesting that milk is actually quite an inefficient means of obtaining the associated nutrients, in this case because so much fluid has to be consumed to absorb the required amounts of those nutrients.

* * * * * * *

It is actually quite interesting that we consider cows' milk to be 'natural' for us, when so many of us would consider it to be unusual for older children to consume their own mother's milk after about two years of age. That sort of thing is even the subject of television programmes on the 'weird and wonderful' of our society. Nor would we probably like the idea of consuming milk from a pig, cat, dog or any other animal, and most of us would probably not relish the thought of consuming cows' milk directly from the udder (or at least if there are people who think that is normal, the 'weird and wonderful' TV lot have yet to get their cameras on them).

Once delivered to our doors in shiny glass bottles, or viewed in row upon row in the supermarket, we have been sterilised to the reality of it all and take it to be entirely normal and natural. Stone Age society and its influences have been critical to our survival as a species, but modern society is such a peculiar thing. Do we really require scientific evidence to understand something that should be so 'obvious'? Culture clearly has a lot to answer for here, because there is no other reason we would have taken to dairy – as a society – in the way we have.

There are no benefits to dairy consumption that cannot be better derived through consumption of green leafy vegetables, sweet potatoes and dark fish. However, there are potential costs of dairy consumption, including an increased risk of cardiovascular disease, stroke, and some cancers. Milk of any kind is simply not required after weaning, and the habit of recommending dairy products for bone health is clearly out-of-date and inaccurate. However, a minimal intake of dairy is likely to be insufficient to cause harm, so those who cannot get through Christmas without Stilton, or a daily tea or coffee without milk, should not panic. Having stated this, there are numerous benefits of teas and coffees, which become limited when the absorption of important nutrients is inhibited by the presence of milk. We can have a little dairy if we like, but should have it in moderate or small amounts and because we like it, rather than because it is still commonly thought of as beneficial.

An Introduction to Bone Health

"The...patient should be made to understand that he or she must take charge of his own life. Don't take your body to the doctor as if he were a repair shop."

- Quentin Regestein

Bone is made up of two key components: the matrix and the minerals. The matrix is the network of scaffolding, made mostly of proteins, and the mineral building blocks are deposited upon that matrix. So, the matrix gives bones their shape and flexibility, whilst the minerals create the rigidity. During early life, children require a good amount of protein to support the development of their bones, but throughout the rest of life it is the *turnover* of bone that is most important.

All cells in the body have their own lifecycles, with their own genetically predetermined generation, functioning and death. In bones, the process of replacing old bone with new is referred to as bone turnover, so old bone material is removed and new minerals replace them, ensuring that bone remains healthy. From an evolutionary perspective, we humans are one of very few species who actually live for a long time after our reproductive age has ended, but there is an important difference between living longer and being healthy throughout life. As we have historically been less active in old age (based upon our observations of modern hunter-gatherer societies), there were never evolutionary pressures to grow old gracefully, as all that was important was growing old. So, although we became good at growing old, we never became good at doing it well, and biologically we do suffer with age, giving us more to do to remain healthy and avoid diseases, such as osteoporosis.

As a species we survived better because older people were around to help at the homestead with the young children, but if one grandparent hobbled a bit where another was more physically capable, this difference would have gone unnoticed, genetically at least. Nowadays these effects are still present. We are able to live to an old age, and women can live for longer after their menopause than they lived before it, which from a biological perspective is astonishing. But it is not easy to age well. We have to work hard because our genetic capacity is limited, and the only way to compensate for this is by influencing the environmental factors – remaining physically active and ensuring we have all the nutrients we need to help prevent the age-related mental and physical declines. As we grow older, bone material is broken down far more readily than it is replaced, leading to fragility and weakness.

From birth our bones grow and develop, becoming longer, thicker and more densely mineralised, and once they have reached their peak – known as our peak bone mass – the bones gradually lose their mineral content, as the turnover system loses efficiency and more bone is removed than is replaced. The bones later become more brittle, and there is an increased risk that they will fracture following an impact.

* * * * * * *

Osteoblasts are the cells responsible for building the bone matrix and depositing minerals within it, whereas osteoclasts dig pits in the bone to remove the older material so it can be replaced by the osteoblasts. During growth the osteoblasts are more active than the osteoclasts, so there is a net gain in bone material at that time. Later on – typically during the twenties and early thirties – the activity of osteoblasts and osteoclasts is more balanced, and bone density and quality is maintained. As we grow older, the osteoclasts become more active than the osteoblasts, and the bones begin to lose density. This in itself is perhaps over-simplistic, owing to the influences of diet and exercise that can affect the balance in either direction, but generally this is the trend observed.

Bone is so much more than an accumulation of minerals upon a structural matrix. In an ideal world we would have a good understanding of what specific factors of bone contribute the most to fractures, so that interventions can be better tested and developed to reduce fracture risk. For example, is the level of mineralisation most important, the rate of remodelling, properties of the matrix itself, occurrence and severity of damage on the smallest level, the mineral density or something else?[136]

As it happens, bone mineral density is the most commonly used marker of bone health, but this is not because it is the most useful thing to measure, but rather because it is the *easiest* thing to measure. An indication of mineralisation and mineral loss can be estimated at a given moment in time from blood and urine tests, but these are very indirect and are meaningful only at the moment the samples were taken. Five minutes later it all might have changed.

Traditional thinking has been that, because bone loss increases with age, the higher our peak bone mass during growth, the further bone mineral density will have to fall before osteoporosis and increased fracture risk occur. This has led to recommendations and efforts to increase childhood and adolescent physical activity levels and calcium intake, in the belief these factors will maximise peak bone mass, thereby increasing the number of years of old age before bone mass and density has fallen enough to be a health concern.

As discussed, bone quality is dependent upon both genetic and environmental factors. We are genetically programmed to have a certain bone mineral density and bone quality, and this can be augmented by diet and weight-bearing exercise. An individual can work very hard to increase their bone density at any stage of life, whether that be in childhood or old age, and the bones will respond and bone mineral density and bone quality will increase (although the response is much reduced in old age, but exists in any case). So, an individual increases his or her bone density above the level programmed by their genetics, in much the same way that a bodybuilder can increase his or her muscle size above what was genetically predetermined for them, and both would occur through a specific exercise approach and close attention to dietary factors. Once those environmental factors (diet and exercise) have returned to more normal levels, regardless of whether the original effect resulted in increased bone mass or increased muscle mass, everything will return to the level programmed by genetics. It might take a while for this to happen, but there is currently good evidence to show that increasing bone mass – whether peak bone mass or bone mass at any other period in life – will not have long-lasting effects[137].

This is not to say that people should not bother with exercise during their youth, but rather that we need to be realistic about what is achievable and how long effects last. Physical activity during youth is important for the health of the whole body, as it is at any other time in life. The important approach for bone health is weight-bearing exercise throughout later life, along with a diet favouring a low salt intake and a high intake of fruits and vegetables, so it is less acidic than most modern westernised diets (to be discussed in the next chapter).

Interest is increasing in the use of mineral water to supply the body with a potentially rich source of minerals important for bone health. The calcium in mineral water is highly bioavailable – at least by comparison to milk[138]. A mineral water with a high calcium content will also have either a high sodium or bicarbonate content. Sodium will increase calcium excretion whereas bicarbonate will not. Bicarbonate is an alkali mineral that is actually more important for bone health than calcium[139]. Therefore, mineral waters with a high bicarbonate and calcium content should be preferred over others. An alkali mineral water, rich in bicarbonate, is of greater benefit to bone health than an acidic mineral water high in calcium[140]. Researchers are now claiming there is an urgent need for studies further exploring the effects of fruits and vegetables on bone health and fracture risk[141], due to the effects these foods have on our acid-base balance, and the critical importance of this for bone health.

Acid-Base Balance & Bone Health

"Yet this is health: to have a body functioning so perfectly
that when its few simple needs are met
it never calls attention to its own existence."

-Bertha Stuart Dyment

The acid-base balance of the body is of fundamental importance to human health. How efficiently a cell can work will be affected if the fluid within it becomes too acidic or too alkali. Normal processes ensure the pH of the arterial blood is maintained at a level of 7.4 and venous blood at about 7.36[142]. Whenever the blood pH rises (becomes more alkali or 'base') or lowers (becomes more acidic), the body responds to bring the pH back to normal. What 'normal' is varies in different tissues of the body, with the stomach being highly acidic and regions of the gut being very alkali. The blood and most cells are neutral or slightly alkali.

The 7.4 pH of the blood helps ensure the cells maintain their normal pH. The reactions that take place within cells can be affected by deviations in pH (and temperature, for that matter), which can slow or even stop normal processes. By maintaining a normal pH of the blood – and therefore the pH of the fluids surrounding our tissues – cells can perform their normal actions as they should, which would be compromised if the pH of the blood experienced a chronic change.

Blood acid-base balance relies upon the effective movement of waste chemicals from the blood to the lungs where they can be exhaled, or to the kidneys for elimination in the urine. Because of the involvement of the kidneys in removing acids, urine is usually acidic, but to what degree will vary according to diet and other influences. Research has shown that modern westernised diets are net acid producing, and cause an acid load on the body[143].

With chronic disorders of kidney function, or where metabolic processes consistently increase the acidity of the blood, this can have serious consequences for overall health, particularly relating to bone health[144]. A high acid load increases the risk of kidney stone formation, osteoporosis[145] and hypertension[146]. However, the lungs, kidneys and other systems normally ensure that blood and cellular pH is maintained within very narrow, healthy limits[147].

In the normal, healthy kidney, an increased acid load on the blood leads to increased acidity of the urine. If urinary excretion of acid is insufficient to maintain the blood at a normal pH, then bone can be involved in the buffering process, and calcium can be lost[148]. Importantly, although calcium is lost from the body and calcium is mostly stored in the bones, it is bicarbonate, sodium and potassium that are mostly buffering the blood. Preventing osteoporosis and promoting bone health should therefore be less focussed on increasing calcium intake, and instead on ensuring the diet is less acidic – via a high intake of fruits and vegetables – and that weight-bearing activity is recommended to promote bone strength and density.

* * * * * * *

A recent study concluded that acid load on the body is related to three main factors: 1) the net acid load of the diet, 2) the age-related decline in kidney function, and 3) the amount of dietary sodium chloride (salt). The last point relates to the unusually high amounts of salt we add to our foods nowadays, which is at odds with the low-salt diet we experienced during all our millions of years of evolution and up until very recently. For people consuming a typical, westernised diet, a high salt intake independently increases the risk of kidney stones and osteoporosis[143], in addition to the net acid load already mentioned[145]. Whenever acid load increases (or base load decreases), the kidneys compensate by increasing acid losses in the urine[338].

Short-term, subtle deviations in blood pH are not a problem, but chronically loading the blood with acid-producing foods is cause for concern (as would be chronically loading the blood with alkali foods). There are a multitude of potential causes of systemic acidosis, although most common and serious would be kidney or respiratory disease. Other potential causes include anaerobic exercise[*], gastroenteritis, *excessive* consumption of protein or other acidifying substances, diabetes, anaemias, AIDS, ageing, and the menopause [142]. Acidosis can also occur locally as a result of increased metabolic activity within a cell, vascular disease, ischaemia, inflammation, infection, tumours, wounds and fractures.

Calcium has historically been understood to have a role in buffering the blood from an acidic pH to a neutral one. Because 99% of the calcium in the body is stored within the bones, it has long been believed that anything that promotes acidity of the blood will increase the release of calcium out of the bones.

Following an acidifying stress on the blood urinary calcium excretion will increase[144], indicating it has *probably* been released from its storage sites in bone[149]. However, it is not the only mineral of interest/concern, as bicarbonate is also lost[144]. Further, despite the assumptions, there is actually no good quality evidence that the calcium lost comes from bone[150] and not cells or from what was already in the blood. The buffering effect that occurs when an

---

[*] i.e., heavy weight training, sprinting, or any other physical activity involving very high intensity exercise or prolonged breath-holding

acidifying stress affects the blood is twelve-times greater than could be expected based upon calcium release alone, indicating there are other, far greater, factors involved[151]. So, whether the calcium in urine has come from bone, cells or the blood directly is only of trivial interest, as there is a greater loss of other bone minerals to buffer an acid load, and this is of far greater relevance to bone health. Calcium is involved in buffering an acid load, but its origins are uncertain and effects fairly minimal.

* * * * * * *

The activity of the pit-digging osteoclasts is dependent upon acidity levels outside the cells. Osteoclasts have been found to be inactive at a pH above 7.3, but are maximally stimulated at a pH of 6.9. Even changes as slight as 0.05 can cause a doubling or halving of bone pit formation[152]. Severe systemic acidosis (pH decrease of about -0.05 to -0.2) often results from renal disease. A milder, chronic acidosis (pH change of about -0.02 to -0.05), can be caused by the more common factors already mentioned, such as excessive protein intake, prolonged exercise, ageing, or the menopause[152].

Cell function, including that of the bone-building osteoblasts, is normally impaired by acid. The unusual stimulatory effect of acid on osteoclasts may represent a primitive 'fail-safe', which evolved with terrestrial vertebrates to correct acidosis, by causing the release of alkaline bone mineral when the lungs and kidneys were unable to maintain the right pH. Even very subtle (but prolonged) acidosis could be sufficient to cause appreciable bone loss over time[152].

An acid load on the body does not only increase the release of alkali minerals from the bones, but also decreases activity of the bone building osteoblasts too[153,154]. Ageing is involved because the kidneys become less able to remove excess acids, meaning a greater reliance is placed upon the bone minerals to compensate for this[154].

So, the first thing we need to do is forget about calcium in particular, because it is *all* alkaline bone minerals that have the potential to be removed. In short, the pH of the blood is maintained primarily via the functions of the lungs and kidneys, and when this is insufficient the alkali substances leaving bones and cells can also contribute. When the blood is acidic, osteoclast activity increases whilst the activity of the bone-building osteoblasts comes to a halt. Conversely, at a more neutral or alkali pH, the reverse is true.

There are regional differences in the response of bone to a chronic acid load. Phosphate is lost from the cross-section of bone, whereas bicarbonate is lost from the bone surface [155]. Further, it is not only those minerals that are used to buffer an acid load. A study published in the *Journal of Bone Mineral Research*[156] reported that other material within bone – the sodium and potassium – is also responsible for buffering an acid load on the blood, rather than the minerals themselves. This is in agreement with the findings of an earlier paper[157], in which it was commented that calcium losses would have to be substantial to buffer an acid load, whereas the release of bicarbonate, sodium and potassium is far more significant[157].

In response to an acid load, bone sodium, potassium, phosphate and bicarbonate are all involved in the buffering process, supporting the idea that bone buffers changes in pH through a number of mechanisms[158]. Additional acid buffering comes from any alkali substances leaving other cells[159], and other substances in the blood, carried by haemoglobin and proteins[142].

Many of us regularly consume high protein foods – such as meats and fish – which is perfectly fine to a point, as such proteins are important for health and those foods contain many essential fats, minerals and other nutrients. The problem is that many people also tend consume a high amount of cereal grains, such as breakfast cereals, bread and pasta, in addition to dairy foods. These contain a combination of carbohydrates and proteins (and fats in the case of dairy), but they contribute a net acid load on the body, as do the meats and fish.

In our ancient diets, we would have obtained all our carbohydrates from fruits and vegetables, which have an alkalising effect on the blood, and could buffer the effects of meat and fish. However, the modern westernised diet has substituted about 80% of the carbohydrates that would originally have been fruits and vegetables with cereal grains and dairy products. So, whereas we would have buffered a reasonable intake of acidifying foods with fruits and vegetables, we have not only reduced our intake (and therefore buffering capacity), but compounded the problem by substituting those fruits and vegetables with more acid-producing foods. This has meant a reasonable intake of both acid-producing and base-producing foods has been exchanged for a diet largely comprised of acid-producing ones.

Interestingly, long-term *non-excessive* protein intake (around 35% of total energy intake) actually increases bone mineral density, possibly through an increased absorption of calcium in the gut, and a preferential effect on metabolic hormone levels. Although a high protein diet increases the acidity of urine and its ammonium content (a by-product of protein metabolism), neither a high nor low protein intake leads to the development of a clinically detectable acidosis by itself[160]. The first thought is that normal kidney and respiratory processes prevent the acidosis from occurring, and the second thought is that even a high protein intake is not necessarily sufficient to be the *excessive* intake required to cause problems in healthy individuals.

A study which compared a high-protein but low-sodium, base-producing diet with a high-carbohydrate, low-fat diet[55], reported that it was the subjects in the high carbohydrate, low-fat group who exhibited the highest rate of bone turnover (increased osteoclast activity). Those in the high meat group had low calcium losses in the urine, which is likely to be beneficial for long-term bone health[55]. However, the positive findings in the meat group were not associated with meat itself, but the fact the diet was low in sodium and was base-producing overall. So, the focus is not to restrict protein intake *per se*, but to ensure there is a balance between intakes of proteins and base-producing foods, with the focus being to ensure the diet is low in salt and high enough in fruits and vegetables to buffer dietary acids.

* * * * * * *

In order to restore a fully natural diet that is bone-healthy, we would need to replace cereal grains and dairy foods with fruits and vegetables. There is now growing interest in the concept that the most appropriate alternative therapy for treating osteoporosis is a diet high in these more natural sources of carbohydrate[141]. The findings of another recent investigation[150] concluded that a high-protein intake with sufficient calcium, fruits and vegetables was important for bone health and the prevention of osteoporosis.

Alkaline therapies correct abnormal bone cell functions and increase bone mineral density, including in patients whose kidneys do not function correctly[161]. Metabolic alkalosis[*] increases influx of calcium into bone[158]. However, chronic alkalosis still takes the blood away from its normal pH, so although beneficial for bone health there would be adverse consequences on other tissues. The most appropriate recommendation is to focus on a balanced diet, naturally high in proteins from meats and fish, high in fruits and vegetables, and low in salt, which will promote a neutral pH, prevent acidosis and support bone health.

---

[*] Alkalosis is the opposite of acidosis, and occurs when the blood is chronically alkali. This could be caused by too much bicarbonate in the blood.

Hydration

*"The only way to keep your health is to eat what you don't want,
drink what you don't like, and do what you'd rather not."*

- Mark Twain

There are various arguments we tend to hear regarding why we ought to focus our attentions on hydration. They usually begin with some background information on just how much of us is water. So as to avoid disappointing anyone, we can do the same here. How much water we contain varies according to our body composition and gender. A lean man will comprise a little more water than a lean woman, with around 60% and 55%, respectively (these figures will vary widely depending upon age and various other factors). People who carry more muscle will have a greater percentage of their weight as water (towards 75%), whereas people who carry more fat will have a lower water percentage (down to 45%).

Of that water, two-thirds is contained within our cells as intra-cellular fluid (ICF). The remaining third is the extra-cellular fluid (ECF), which is everything else. The extra-cellular fluid includes blood (20% of total ECF), and the interstitial fluid – the fluid that surrounds cells and acts as the medium between the blood and the cell, where all the nutrients, gases and other substances are exchanged. Oxygen and nutrients pass from the blood into the interstitial fluid before reaching the cells, and carbon dioxide and waste products leave the cells into the interstitial fluid before entering the blood. The fluids contained with the lymphatic system, surrounding the brain and spine, within joints, and all the other fluid regions make up the 80% of ECF that is not blood, including fluids in the eyes and ears.

So, water is everywhere; it is the liquid portion of the blood (the rest being cells, nutrients, immune factors and so on), it bathes the cells and acts as a medium between the cells and the blood, it protects the brain and spinal cord, is part of the lymphatic system and supports our joints. Within the cells, water is the medium through which chemical reactions occur, and is an important component of some reactions and a by-product of others. How much water is within the cells, blood, and interstitial fluid is tightly controlled and dependent upon the concentration of other substances present, such as sodium and potassium.

Part of the control of water balance occurs within and around the cells themselves, but on a whole-body scale the kidneys manage this, with additional influences from the heart and brain. If we have an insufficient water intake, the kidneys ensure that much of the fluid entering them is secreted back into the blood, causing urine to be low in volume and highly concentrated in waste products. Similarly, if sodium concentrations are too high, more sodium is lost in the urine so it becomes more concentrated. Conversely, if we consume too much water our urine becomes high in volume and dilute, with a lower concentration of sodium being lost. All this is to maintain total body water balance.

The heart is involved because nerves detect fluctuations in blood pressure. If there is a high or low volume of fluid in the blood, this will affect blood pressure and the heart will detect the changes. The nerves pass the signal to the brain, which then signals the kidneys to lose or retain water accordingly. Coinciding with this, the hypothalamus in the brain will initiate feelings of thirst or satiety accordingly. Similarly, if there is too much water or too little sodium, the brain will trigger a desire for salty foods. In addition to the heart's pressure sensors, there are also chemical sensors that keep a check on the composition of the blood. This demonstrates there is a multifaceted and complex homeostatic regulation of hydration, co-ordinated primarily by the kidneys but further supported by the heart and brain through a highly developed network of sensors and signallers. What we might notice is simply a desire to drink or not to drink, a desire to consume or avoid salty foods, and perhaps we will see changes in the concentration of our urine (clear or coloured, according to the concentration of waste products).

So, where does this leave those who like to dictate that a conscious effort is required to consume a specific amount of water each day? There certainly seem to be plenty of websites and individuals adamant we need two litres a day, or some other amount based upon complicated estimations from bodyweight. Well, having evolved within and surrounded by a fluid environment, over a period of some few thousand million years, it is fair to say that we – like all other living organisms, whether mammalian, amphibian, reptilian, bacterial or whatever else – have had plenty of time to evolve our inherent, homeostatic regulatory systems for managing water balance. Our kidneys, unless very seriously damaged, manage this to a very high standard, and as long as we do not ignore our internal cues for food and water for too long we will do just fine. Despite what some might like us to think, we cannot easily improve upon thousands of millions of years of adaptation. All we have to do – and this point cannot be stressed strongly enough – is eat and drink whenever we have the desire to do so, and everything will then be just fine.

There are exceptions to this, such as in athletes during exercise, because when engaged in dehydrating exercise the thirst mechanism is not as effective as we would like it to be, mostly on account of an evolutionary history of being moderately physically active, rather than intensely physically active. As this is relevant only to a very small percentage of the population, it is a discussion for elsewhere. For those who really are interested there is a respectably in-depth review of hydration for athletes in my book on *The Jungle Marathon*, although much of the information is freely available on my website.

Suffice it to state, however, that many of the problems athletes suffer from are actually related to over-consumption of water and/or over- or under-consumption of salts. This is actually not because the system is inherently inefficient, but because people attempt to prevent dehydration by over-ruling their actual desires for foods and fluids, consume water and processed powders at a rate the body cannot respond to fast enough, and suffer problems as a result. Dehydration alone typically reduces performance, reduces co-ordination and means more has to be done afterwards to compensate. The real problems come when people try to second-guess their requirements and consciously go to great lengths that end up being destructive. This has been covered elsewhere, however, and for the majority of readers there is no need to go deeper into this here. Another exception would be for those in certain disease states, but their doctor or specialist would already have given them the most appropriate advice.

So, is there an amount of water we do need to take in each day? Well, we gain water via the consumption of fluids, foods and the production of water as a by-product of cellular reactions. We lose water mostly in the urine, via evaporation through the skin (either as sweat or unnoticeable perspiration), via our breath as we exhale and through the intestines as faecal waste. Ingested liquids contribute roughly 1600-millilitres of our water 'gain', with foods providing about another 700-ml of fluid, and metabolic reactions producing about 200-ml. Conversely, the kidneys lose about 1500-ml a day, with a further 600-ml being lost through the skin, 300-ml via the lungs, and about 100-ml via the intestines.

This makes approximately 2.5 litres of water gain matching about 2.5 litres of water loss. If it is a hot day and more water is lost in sweat, then we will feel more thirsty and want to have more fluids to drink, or else to eat foods with a high fluid content (such as many types of fruits and vegetables). However, if we drink more than we need then fairly soon we will lose the desire to drink, and urine output will increase. If we eat a lot of salty foods we will feel thirsty and our urine will contain a high concentration of salt and only a little water.

So, in terms of total quantity of fluid intake, there is really no point whatsoever in attempting to measure, gauge or in any way analyse what this should be (unless a disease state or disorder is present, which happens to mean the body's natural systems are not working properly). For most of us, we simply need to drink when we are thirsty. To measure fluid intake is meaningless unless we are measuring the fluid contribution from foods too, and analysing in advance what the metabolic water production would be. Fluid 'requirements' are far too complex to analyse with any degree of accuracy on a daily basis. Fortunately, our wonderful brains have evolved to be highly effective at giving us simple messages we can understand relating to this. As long as we do not ignore any such internal cues for too many hours or days, we ought to be just fine.

Is there any specific type of fluid we ought to consume in preference to others? Well, we can drink mineral water if we choose, or fruit smoothies, or tea, or coffee or gin. Genuinely, any liquid we consume will contribute to our total fluid intake. Caffeinated drinks and alcohol sometimes get a bad press because they have a 'diuretic' effect, meaning they encourage urine losses above what would be expected for the amount of fluid consumed. However, even though this is true, the total amount lost is still less than that consumed, meaning there is a net gain. There might be other reasons to avoid too much coffee, alcohol, fruit juice and soft drinks, but hydration is not one of them.

For whatever reason there are people who attempt to over-complicate the matter of hydration. The actual homeostatic, hormonal and nervous control of water balance is highly complicated, but the actual result of that inherent complexity is that the body manages itself far more efficiently than some people like to think.

Water is the substance of life, and because of this we have become incredibly effective and efficient at keeping it in balance. Just as lions, antelopes and crocodiles can get by without being told when, what and how much to drink, so can we. For those of us who engage in physical activity in a manner that is different to that experienced during our evolutionary past, the system whilst exercising is less efficient, but when we come to rest normal functioning is rapidly resumed. For all of us, that dryness we get in the mouth on a warm day or when we have not had a drink for a while – this is not a coincidence – it is a biological, evolutionary effect that acts as one prompt amongst many that we need to increase our fluid levels. So when we feel thirsty we ought to have a glass of mineral water, a smoothie, some fruit or a cup of tea – I mean, why not – if we feel like we want some why avoid the urge? Really, how complicated does it need to be?

Water

*"I never drink water because of the disgusting things
that fish do in it."*

- W. C. Fields

Mineral Water

There are those who scoff at the very concept of mineral water. This
is traditionally on the basis that tap water is so much cheaper and,
when it comes down to it, it is all just water anyway. Really the
debate should be focussed on the benefits of mineral waters for the
health of the bones and cardiovascular system, and the health
consequences of consuming too much water containing potentially
harmful substances.

A high magnesium and bicarbonate content in mineral water
has been associated with less acidic urine (suggesting reduced acid
persisting in the blood), and a reduced risk of kidney stone formation
[162]. The magnesium in mineral water has been shown to have a
bioavailability at least as high as that of good food sources of the
mineral[163]. Other researchers have reported that magnesium from
mineral waters cannot be taken in excess, as the kidneys are effective
at removing any of the mineral that is superfluous[164]. Interestingly,
the use of mineral water containing a varied concentration of minerals,
including a high amount of magnesium, has been shown to
significantly decrease blood pressure[165].

The absorption of calcium should be much higher from

mineral waters compared with other sources. This is because calcium absorption decreases as more is taken in, but mineral water can be taken in small amounts throughout the day, maximising the potential for total calcium intake into the blood[166]. Although calcium is important for bone health, other minerals – such as bicarbonate – are even more useful due to their positive effects on reducing bone mineral losses[167]. Hence, recommendations to increase mineral water intake should not be based on the calcium content alone, but rather on the contribution of all the minerals to bone health, particularly for the more alkali waters[167].

Unlike normal drinking water, natural mineral water has to be bottled as it is, without any interference to alter the bacterial content. Because of the lifecycle of natural mineral water, it is to be expected that it contains a rich spectrum of bacteria, and the bottling process does not appear to affect them. In fact, the number of bacteria increases dramatically once within the bottle, and this has been demonstrated by comparing the bacterial content at the source and then a few weeks after bottling[168]. Interestingly, none of the bacteria found in that study were related in any way to bacteria known to be harmful. Although this investigation did not analyse every mineral water currently available, and its testing was only at a single point in time, it certainly supports the idea that mineral waters are perfectly safe to consume. Rigorous testing of mineral waters is required to ensure safety standards are met, and any potentially harmful bacteria are detected at source.

So, water contains a rich source of bacteria, which may either be of benefit or have no consequence to the human body. Further, the minerals may directly buffer any acidity in the blood, and such minerals may also be available to be taken up into the bones to contribute to bone mineral content and quality. Mineral water has also been found to reduce blood pressure in individuals with hypertension.

* * * * * * *

There are concerns regarding the packaging of food items and drinks in plastic containers, due to the risks that chemicals within the plastics can leach out into the food or drink, where they might then have the capacity to do harm. Some of these chemicals can act as hormone-disruptors, with the potential to increase levels of the sex hormone oestrogen. Even when such chemicals do produce an observable effect, there needs to be some consideration of whether or not the effect would be a negative one in humans. Other unwanted chemicals could potentially harm cells and organs directly, although the concentrations of these tend to be so low that any real risk is unlikely.

Hormone levels fluctuate naturally during the course of the day, and a very small increase in oestrogen is unlikely to have any physiological effect worthy of concern. However, should hormone levels be affected adversely on a daily basis, there is reason to be sceptical about consuming any fluids from plastic bottles, and the concerns would be greatest for children and adolescents. Plastic bottles manufactured using PET (polyethylene terephthalate) are of particular interest in this regard, and it is the phthalic acid and related chemicals that are associated with a potential to cause harm.

A recent Italian study[169] reported that in more than 90% of mineral waters tested, there was no appreciable oestrogen-promoting activity, although amongst the samples they did find very low concentrations of these substances. Levels of hormone-disrupting chemicals have been found to be about 20-times higher in plastic bottles than glass ones[170]. However, the investigators referred to here did not find any indication that the chemicals had any effect on consumers. This finding conflicts with a study published a year after theirs, in which it was found that endocrine disruptors do have the capacity to affect human hormone levels[171].

In addition to phthalic acid and its related chemicals, aldehyde and other substances can also be transferred from the plastic bottles into the mineral water[172]. Another Italian study[173] reported that many still and sparkling mineral waters contained chemicals from the plastic bottles that could damage DNA, and suggested that as well as direct transfer from the plastic bottles, the plastic pipelines that transported the water could also contribute. When it comes to water transported along plastic pipes, this raises a similar need to gather research on those same chemicals in tap water.

The movement of chemicals from the plastic into mineral water will be influenced by temperature, duration of storage, concentrations of the specific chemicals within the bottle, the pH of the water, and the concentration of carbon dioxide gas in the water[172]. The effects of low levels of these substances on something as big as the human body appear to be negligible, but it would be good practice not to store mineral waters for extended periods, especially once opened. Direct sunlight and high temperatures should be avoided, still water should be preferred over sparkling, and alkaline mineral waters (already of greatest benefit to bone health) should be favoured over more acidic ones.

The main issue is not that mineral water is bad because it is commonly stored in plastic bottles, but rather that more needs to be done to avoid the use of such plastics in *all* food and fluid storage. As consumers, by choosing to purchase products in glass and other packaging, we can reduce the amount of these potentially harmful substances we are being exposed to. When we do buy food and drink in plastic containers, it would be preferable to transfer the items into more robust containers for storage.

A study published over ten years ago[174] called for both more information on the composition of mineral waters, and detailing of the effects of mineral concentrations that were particularly high or low. Labels on mineral water bottles do include some information regarding their composition, although it could be of more use to consumers if more information were included. A pH close to 7.4, a high bicarbonate and calcium content, and a low sodium content, would all be beneficial for bone health.

The transfer of chemicals from plastic pipes prior to bottling is interesting, particularly when we consider how far tap water travels before reaching the tap. Should evidence emerge to demonstrate that a genuine risk exists, then the safest reasonable option is mineral water bottled at source into glass containers. However, the likelihood is the levels of such contaminants from plastic pipes are extremely low. Any effects to human physiology would be of such miniscule proportions as to be overshadowed by natural hormone fluctuations throughout the day. Perhaps there would be greater issue if we were exposing ourselves to numerous contaminants, with them having an accumulating effect on the body. On balance though, consuming plenty of pH-neutral or slightly alkaline mineral water, high in bicarbonate and calcium, and low in sodium, has far more benefits than other waters, most notably for cardiovascular and bone health.

Tap Water

Tap water is, for the most part, perfectly safe and the water of choice for most of us. There are clear benefits to mineral water, and overall a mineral water should certainly be healthier than tap water, but in and of itself tap water is typically acceptable. There is an urban myth about tap water having passed through however many people (seven or thereabouts) before reaching us, but assigning such numbers is ludicrous. Water has been on this planet – whether in solid, liquid or gas form – for thousands of millions of years. It is not mystically recycled out in space, and the water we consume – whether mineral water, spring water or tap water – has likely passed through the digestive systems of millions of organisms before it reaches our mouths. The concern is really not that H_2O itself has been around for a long time before we get to drink it – because hydrogen and oxygen are simply atoms and cannot therefore be clean, unclean or contaminated – it is the issue of what comes *with* our H_2O.

The problem is that the water coming from our taps is not simply H_2O – it is H_2O *plus* all the other substances that might have been in wherever the water was sourced from. In most large cities the water is sourced from rivers, and those rivers could be full of biological waste products (from fish down to bacteria) as well as chemicals from industry, agriculture and human waste. What goes into the water treatment plants is certainly not just H_2O, but what we need to consider is if there is anything that might actually do harm, and whether or not this is managed by elimination (via filtering), reduction (via chemical reactions with added substances), or is simply checked upon to ensure it remains within safe limits.

With mineral water the expectation is that filtering has occurred naturally – through various layers and depths of rocks – and it emerges for bottling clean enough that no further filtering or processing is required. Tap water, by contrast, can come from river sources that might contain not only industrial, agricultural and environmental waste, but wastewater from human sewage systems as well. Hence, public drinking water is heavily filtered, but there is always a risk of contamination from any of the waste sources. Mostly, these are kept well within what are considered to be safe limits, but whether or not a high consumption of tap water from a particular region might carry the potential for harm, particularly to young children, is a complex and involved topic.

The Colorado River in the US has been contaminated by a chemical called ammonium perchlorate, which is an industrial and agricultural waste product. Although the effects of this chemical are still debated[175,176], even low levels of this contaminant in drinking water have been associated with thyroid disorders in newborns[177], even as recently as 2010[178]. However, another study reported the average exposure of Americans to this chemical is now lower than it used to be[179], and one study published over a decade previously[180] reported no association between the drinking water in California and thyroid problems in newborns. Differences in findings could be explained by regional fluctuations, fluctuations over time, or improvements in measuring techniques.

The disinfectants used to prepare water for human consumption, although safe themselves, have been reported to generate potentially harmful by-products[181]. Some chemicals thought to be responsible for contributing to feminisation of exposed fish have also been reported in drinking water. These hormone disrupters (oestrogen-promoters, to be more specific) may occur during water treatment and subsequently interfere with human hormone levels[182]. This finding was the result of a study in the UK, although recent studies in France[183], Germany[184], and the US[107,185], have also reported oestrogen promoters in rivers and wastewater treatment plants.

All those studies reported the presence of hormone-disrupting chemicals in drinking water, which arrived there having passed through sewage treatment plants. However, that these chemicals can have significant effects on human health is not conclusive, with some investigators reporting no effects in humans[186]. Again, there may be fluctuations according to where the water is sourced from, the year and time of year, and differences due to technologies used in measuring.

The author of an Australian research paper[187], alluded to the fact the water in the River Thames in London passes through drinking water and sewage discharge five times before reaching the end of the Thames estuary. Here, as in many other highly populated countries and regions, the sewage is emptied into the same water supply from which the drinking water is sourced.

Drinking water also contains nitrates, which in high levels can negatively impact on human health. The amount of nitrate in drinking water has increased over past decades due to contamination of water from fertilizers, animal and human waste, legume crops, and industrial waste[188]. Although nitrates in foods are a concern for our health, the amounts in drinking water are usually very low, and typically protected against by our intake of fruits and vegetables[188].

Unwanted chemicals in drinking water typically vary by location. Lithium has been detected in the water from the Andes mountains in Argentina, which could have adverse affects on the thyroid function of consumers[189]. The Colorado river was mentioned earlier as a site of perchlorate contamination, but it has also recently been reported to have a high concentration of uranium due to local mining[190]. Uranium is another oestrogen-promoting substance, which can increase the risk of fertility problems and reproductive cancers[190].

For the most part, however, the concentration of unwanted chemicals in drinking water is extremely low and considered to be safe for general consumption. Nitrates can be removed by the use of a reverse-osmolarity filter or steam distilling, and more common water filters can remove some of the larger chemicals. Where water quality is a concern, or if consumption of any level of these contaminants does not appeal, then mineral water is the healthier option. Realistically, a combination of both is probably the most appropriate and convenient middle ground, with mineral water consumed as drinking water and filtered tap water used for hot drinks and cooking.

Teas, Coffee & Health

"Where there's tea, there's hope."

- Arthur W. Pinero

A quick search on Pubmed for research articles with either tea or coffee in the title returns an impressive number of papers. In fact, there is an overwhelming volume of evidence to support the benefits of different teas and coffee. Before detailing this further, there are a few introductory points that ought to be made.

Black tea, green tea, white tea, and coffees all contain caffeine in varying amounts, and caffeine itself is a stimulant. Becoming dependent on caffeine can have negative consequences, in that people become tolerant of caffeine fairly quickly, meaning it then has to be consumed at various points during the day simply to feel 'normal'. The problem here is that quality of life *could* be affected if a person is tired, sleepy and lethargic during periods when they have not recently consumed a tea or coffee. It is not necessarily a problem, because we can readily reduce our intakes if we feel dependent. It is just a point worth making and to consider. Because caffeine dilates blood vessels, withdrawal from normal amounts can cause headaches, although these should disappear when caffeine is consumed again. Should caffeine be having this effect, it is probably best to gradually reduce intake.

The alternative to caffeine dependence is of course to sleep deeply and fully each night, and to ensure we feel good during the day without the need for a stimulant. That ought to be preferable, but other than the potential for dependence there are virtually no downsides at all to caffeine consumption from teas and coffees. In higher doses caffeine can have transient effects on the heart, increasing heart rate and potentially inducing palpitations, but again this is something to be wary of rather than a reason to avoid caffeine-containing drinks (unless specifically recommended to do so on an individual basis by a specialist, obviously). An investigation of the effects of caffeine on the heart actually reported no unfavourable effects on function in healthy adults[191], although blood pressure and heart rate were found to increase transiently.

Caffeine, like alcohol, is a diuretic, meaning it promotes urine loss above that expected for the volume of fluid consumed. However, overall a cup of tea or coffee is still going to promote hydration, because although urine losses might be more than would follow drinking water or a fruit juice, the balance will still be in favour of promoting fluid gain over loss. The strength of the diuretic effect will also depend upon levels of hydration, physical activity, and individual factors, but the detail is not necessary and this is simply to say specific information is unavailable.

For many people living in westernised societies, it is now commonly the case that teas and coffees are either the primary or secondary source of daily fluids, and because the benefits far outweigh the costs for the majority, there is every reason to encourage this. The 'costs' that would tip the balance in favour of avoidance would be sensitivity to caffeine, whereby some individuals are more likely to suffer the effects on the heart or become easily reliant upon it, and potentially negative effects on bone mass – to be discussed later. It should also be noted that many of the studies reporting the benefits and bioavailability of nutrients within teas and coffees, tended to focus on milk-free consumption, as milk could interfere with absorption of many of the important plant chemicals.

Teas and coffees are unusual in that they are a plant food not categorised as either fruit or vegetable, but are rich in anti-oxidant phytochemicals[192]. Teas are particularly rich in flavonoids, including catechins, flavonols, theaflavin and thearubigin[193]. The catechins in green tea confer anti-oxidant properties several times greater than those of vitamins C and E[194].

Black, green and oolong tea all come from the same plant (*Camellia sinensis*), but are processed to different levels. Green tea is fermented into oolong tea and then further into black tea. Green tea itself is processed via drying and treatment with hot steam and air[195,196]. This processing affects the nutrient composition of the teas, but the rich spectrums of nutrients in each type of tea are all beneficial in their own ways [197].

Some of the nutrients in teas have been found to reduce total and LDL cholesterol *in vivo*[193,339], and protect LDL cholesterol against peroxidation *in vitro* (peroxidation of LDL cholesterol has been associated with atherosclerosis)[193]. The mechanism by which tea might protect against heart disease is still unclear[198]. However, that tea consumption confers both short-term and long-term beneficial effects on the health of the cardiovascular system is well-supported, and is associated with reductions in blood pressure[199] and improvements in blood cholesterol profiles and blood vessel health[200].

Both black and green tea consumption have been shown to improve anti-oxidant capacity[201]. Green tea has potent anti-oxidant effects[202], as the plant chemicals can scavenge reactive oxygen and nitrogen species, and prevent metals from foods causing harm[203]. Green tea has also been shown to protect the liver[202], the lining of the intestines[204], and the kidneys[205] from damage. Frequent green tea intake has been found to decrease the formation of dental caries[195].

A recent review[203] discussed the *pro-oxidative* capacity of green tea. As mentioned in the chapter on anti-oxidants, substances can be anti-oxidant or pro-oxidant depending upon the requirements of the cell, and we are still only beginning to understand these relationships and their relevance to human health. Hence, more research is required to further elucidate these properties, although it would be wise to be sceptical of any purported benefits of tea extracts, which are more concentrated than tea itself. The conclusion of an extensive review of research on green tea[195] was that green tea consumption should be promoted, as it is an important, health-promoting drink.

Interestingly, green tea has been found to be higher in anti-oxidant capacity than black tea[206]. Similarly, oolong tea has been shown to have a high anti-oxidant capacity and to promote a feeling of relaxation[207]. Importantly, it is not any one anti-oxidant chemical that is responsible for the overall anti-oxidant capacity, but rather the interactions between lots of the plant chemicals within the tea[206]. The catechins contained within teas have even been shown to destroy malignant cancer cells[208,209].

Research from an American group[210] did find that black tea suppressed the growth of some gut bacteria. In that study, although there was considerable variation in the types of bacteria commonly inhabiting the guts of different subjects, the bacteria that were suppressed by black tea did not belong to any of the groups the researchers were specifically testing for. In other words, a deeper understanding of the types of gut bacteria is necessary before it can be concluded whether the effects of tea on the gut are good or bad. That the bacteria suppressed did not belong to any of the main groups suggests the effects are unlikely to be particularly negative. Another study[211] reported that flavonoids in tea were protective of the gastrointestinal tract, although in agreement with the previous study supported the need for more research to better understand the mechanisms.

The anti-oxidant capacity of black tea has been shown to

protect the liver from damage caused by high-fat diets[212], and inflammation[213]. Tea is also protective against complications associated with diabetes, although this is only one factor amongst many needed to confer overall benefits to the individual[194]. How long the protective effects of any type of tea lasts are still debated[214], indicating more research is required.

Other teas include white tea, which has been found to protect neurons (the cells of the brain and nervous system) from damage [215]. White tea reduces oxidative stress and scavenges ROS and RNS[215]. Rooibos (Red bush, *Aspalathus linearis*) has a high anti-oxidant capacity but is free from caffeine, alkaloids and has a low tannin content[216]. Rooibos has been shown to promote immune function[216] and the anti-oxidants it contains have been shown to protect the liver[217,218] and kidneys from damage[217].

The only real negative of tea is that it has been shown to reduce the absorption of other nutrients, including carbohydrates[197] and fats[196]. It is therefore likely that the absorption of vitamins, minerals and other important nutrients could also be limited by tea consumption. It would therefore be appropriate to avoid drinking tea shortly before, during, or immediately following a meal. Interestingly, although caffeine can have negative effects on bone health, tea itself actually promotes bone health, overall, due to the benefits from the plant chemicals it contains.

* * * * * * *

Caffeine has been shown to increase osteoclast activity[219], and interfere with normal bone processes in rats[220]. One study on rats[221] reported that caffeine increased calcium losses in the urine and led to reduced bone mineral density, and although treadmill exercise slightly reduced the extent of the damage, it did not outweigh the negative effects of caffeine intake on bone health. Despite this, a long-term rat study[222] (140 days) reported that coffee itself did not stimulate bone loss.

The real effects of caffeine intake on the bone health of humans are still debated. One of the reasons is that tea, which for many is not only their main source of caffeine but their main source of fluid too, actually appears to promote bone health, due to its content of bone-supporting phytochemicals, which counteract any negative effects of the caffeine[223]. This is in agreement with similar findings from one of the rat studies previously mentioned[222]. The evidence supports that caffeine has a negative effect on bone health, but tea appears to promote bone health overall, and the effects of coffee are unclear.

Another criticism is that much of the research linking caffeine to osteoporosis was conducted on subjects with very low calcium intakes[224,225] who were already at risk. That a study of rat exercise[221] showed exercise did not compensate for caffeine-induced losses is not representative of exercise in humans, where our two legs, greater mass and greater stresses (weight-for-weight) increase the bone-promoting effects of weight-bearing exercise.

A study of caffeine intake and bone mass among young women[226] (625 women, 14 to 40 years of age) reported there was no overall interaction between caffeine and bone health, with the exception of a reduced bone quality in women using a particular injected contraceptive (DMPA). A similar study[227] reported that normal intakes of caffeine do not affect bone mineral density in 12- to 18-year-old girls.

The same authors[228] found there was no support for the argument that caffeine promotes bone loss in post-menopausal women (aged 55 to 70). However, despite the lack of association between caffeine and bone health in the studies mentioned so far, others have reported negative effects. For example, one study[229] reported that in women aged 65 to 77 years, a caffeine intake greater than 300-mg per day did accelerate bone loss in the spine, and genetic factors increased this in women with a particular trait affecting how their body utilised vitamin D. This amount of caffeine is equivalent to a large mug of brewed coffee from a coffee shop, four shots of espresso, four to six cans of a typical, caffeinated soft drink, or between three and six cups of tea (depending upon type and for how long it was brewed). Energy drinks vary in composition, with 300-mg being the equivalent of one to six servings, depending upon the brand.

Another study[230] (359 men and 358 women, all around 70 years of age) reported that 70-year-old men consuming four or more cups of coffee a day had 4% lower bone mineral density than low or non-consumers of coffee. This difference was not observed in women of the same age, and even in men there were genetic factors that accelerated the negative effects in those with that trait.

Interestingly, studies of caffeine consumption in women[231,232] found that coffee protects against type 2 diabetes, although the mechanisms are unclear[233]. A study of both healthy and diabetic women[234] reported that coffee (caffeinated and de-caffeinated) actually reduced signs of inflammation and blood vessel damage, therefore either preventing harm or supporting health. This is further supported by another study by the same authors[232] who reported that long-term coffee consumption actually decreased risk of stroke in women (sample size of 83,076 women). These findings were associated with coffee specifically, and not tea or caffeinated soft drinks[232].

Other research has focussed upon potential relationships between coffee and cancer, reporting that there is either no association or in some cases a protective effect[235,236]. Coffee consumption has been associated with a reduced breast volume in women with a particular genetic trait, and this relationship has been shown to be protective against breast cancer, although only in women with that specific trait[237].

To summarise, there is an association between caffeine and coffee intake on reduced bone mineral density, although the effects of coffee itself is still debatable and teas themselves are protective. The negative effects found in rat studies have overestimated the association, because in real life the effects of caffeine are usually reduced or prevented entirely due to the phytochemical content of teas and coffees. Importantly, weight-bearing exercise will reduce the effects of caffeine on bone mineral density, although research is required to describe how significant such an effect might be.

Further, it is those of older age (around 70 years) who are at risk, and even then it is those who consume the highest amounts of caffeine (greater than 300-mg per day), and who have a genetic predisposition, who should attempt to reduce coffee consumption. Interestingly, coffee has been shown to support the health of blood vessels, protect against stroke and reduce signs of inflammation. Coffee has also been reported to have either no effect or a protective effect against certain types of cancer, and overall cancer risk in general.

* * * * * * *

The consumption of high-caffeine stimulant drinks for children is a particular and important concern, as there is no reason to suppose the health balance of these tips in any direction but to the negative.

Caffeine consumed along with other stimulants, flavourings, preservatives, and sugars, is not at all comparable to caffeine as a natural component of phytochemical-rich teas and coffees. Research will likely lead to recommendations against the availability of these products to the more vulnerable bodies and minds of children and adolescents. It should also be noted that the research supports consumption of black and green teas directly, and it is more appropriate to consume these rather than the extracts available as herbal remedies, some of which have been found to have negative effects on human health.

There is not really a 'need' for caffeine-rich drinks, although there are unquestionably plenty of benefits of natural products that happen to contain caffeine. The evidence suggests there is every reason to consider teas and coffees as a 'superfood' above all others, simply because of the quantity consumed by the average person. Tea in particular promotes bone health, whilst teas and coffees both promote anti-oxidant capacity, support the health of the blood vessels and reduce inflammation, whilst helping to protect against certain cancers. Further, coffee has been independently shown to protect against type 2 diabetes and stroke.

Tea and coffee consumption should be encouraged as a means to promote nutrient intake, although coffee intake should probably be less than 300-mg a day in people 70 years of age and older. These recommendations should not replace specific advice given on an individual basis by a doctor, particularly to those sensitive to the effects of caffeine. In any case, many herbal and fruit teas – such as rooibos – have beneficial effects and are caffeine-free. De-caffeinated teas and coffees will still contain some caffeine, although the actual concentration will be far lower than caffeinated varieties. Teas and coffees are best taken without milk, so as to promote nutrient absorption, and similarly teas and coffees should not be taken with or immediately before or after meals. This will help ensure we can capitalise on all possible benefits.

> *"There is no trouble so great or grave that cannot be much diminished by a nice cup of tea."*
>> **- Bernard-Paul Heroux**

Supplements

"Our body is a machine for living. It is organized for that, it is its nature. Let life go on in it unhindered and let it defend itself, it will do more than if you paralyze it by encumbering it with remedies."
- Leo Tolstoy

There are three important problems with supplements. The first is that they can be exploitative. The second is that even for a particular supplement from a specific manufacturer, the composition can sometimes vary widely from one batch to the next. The third problem is that the consumer has no way of knowing if the supplement is safe and effective. If there is a negative health effect associated with a supplement, then current legislation is sufficient to allow the manufacturer to have another go at getting it right. Even then, the requirement is only that the supplement is safe – there is absolutely no necessity that the supplement be at all effective. If sufficient unequivocal and unbiased evidence of efficacy were required, then health shops would contain a few vitamin and mineral supplements, some fish oils, a few stimulants and very little else. Manufacturers of natural anti-depressants could make a few reasonable claims, but that would be about it.

In terms of exploitation, the problem here is that the people who tend to take supplements regularly are absolutely not the people with an actual requirement for them. Supplements are more about lifestyle self-image and health aspiration than real need. We seem to love technology so much that if informed we have a nutrient deficiency, rather than enquiring as to which foods we can obtain that nutrient from – or even what the best, most bioaccessible and bioavailable form is – we just want a pill that we imagine is far superior. That is quite an assumption.

A study from a German group[267] found that regular supplement users had healthier diets than non-users, supporting the case that supplements are about health aspiration and lifestyle-image, rather than nutritional deficiencies warranting their use. Of course, some might take them on the assumption they confer benefits above what can be obtained from food, but the reality is that supplementing where it is not required can cause more harm than good. Over-consumption of certain vitamins and minerals can interfere with the absorption of other essential nutrients, promoting deficiencies, and some nutrients become pro-oxidant in high concentrations. Hence, there really is the potential for 'health' supplements – when taken by people without a genuine need – not just to have no effect, but actually to cause harm. That supplements are typically either self-prescribed or recommended from non-experts warrants considerable cause for concern in this regard.

The definition of a nutritional supplement is something that *supplements* the normal diet. If the diet is already sufficient in all regards, then consuming a supplement really can cause problems. Because supplements typically contain nutrients in unusually high concentrations, these can sometimes have a negative effect on health, not just through affecting bioavailability of other nutrients, but by affecting cardiovascular health and hormone balance too.

As has been discussed fairly extensively in the chapter on bone health, calcium is not nearly as important as is traditionally thought. This is because calcium balance is best maintained through a diet rich in green leafy vegetables, sweet potatoes and dark fish. In any case, it is minerals besides calcium that are most important for bone health, such as bicarbonate, phosphate, sodium and potassium.

Further, it has been discussed that calcium intake only has to be above the absolute minimum level, with a greater intake conferring no additional benefits. However, there is still a knee-jerk recommendation that anyone who has or is at risk of osteoporosis should take calcium supplements. But what if too much calcium, taken in a single, high-concentration dose, were actually more harmful to the majority of people advised to take it?

A recent study published in the *British Medical Journal*[268], found that even very low intakes of supplemented calcium (below 500-mg per day) increased risks of cardiovascular events. This is because an increase in blood calcium levels can immediately harm blood vessel walls and increase release of parathyroid hormone, both of which contribute to risk of cardiovascular problems, including heart attacks and stroke[268]. This result has been supported by other studies[269] and a recent meta-analysis[270]

Normally, blood levels of calcium are kept constant, and because a normal meal does not contain very high concentrations of calcium, the intestines adjust absorption as required. A dietary calcium supplement is absorbed too quickly for this protective effect to have a chance to reduce absorption. So, calcium supplements increase risk of heart attacks, stroke and death, and are protective only for the very small proportion of the society who have daily intakes of calcium below the minimum levels. Even for those with very low calcium intakes, who are at risk of osteoporosis and fractures, it would be more appropriate to increase calcium intake through the consumption of fruits, vegetables and small fish rather than supplements, as the high concentrations of calcium in a tablet will increase risk of a cardiovascular event in that population too.

Really, unless someone genuinely cannot obtain sufficient minerals from their diet, there is no reason to consider supplementation. More is more – it is not necessarily better, and sometimes it can actually be a lot worse than the effects of the original deficiency. A diet high in fruits, vegetables, fish and some meat – particularly when combined with regular consumption of a good mineral water – will promote healthy bones and cardiovascular health, whereas a net acid diet with calcium supplements will reduce bone health and increase risk of cardiovascular events. In this regard, supplements are not even a quick-fix: they are a problem, and should only be recommended for individuals with a genuine reason for taking them, where the benefits outweigh the costs, and this should be managed by the appropriate health-care professionals only.

* * * * * * *

The quality of supplements also needs to be questioned. A nutrient manufactured in a laboratory should not be assumed to have greater bioaccessibility and bioavailability than the naturally-occurring equivalent. As has already been discussed, a natural food will be a rich source of perhaps thousands of important phytochemicals, and it is not efficient to manufacture all of these in a laboratory, so only a few are ever included. However, as many nutrients have the greatest effect when present with many others, taking a few synthetically-manufactured chemicals can never really compare to what can be obtained from a healthy, varied diet.

A recent British study[271] found that the quality of raw materials used in the manufacture of nutraceutical supplements varied widely. Importantly, no nutraceutical was found to have a consistently high quality, but many revealed consistently low quality. The lack of adequate regulation was cited as one cause of this problem. Further, the consequences of interactions between different supplements, and between supplements and pharmaceuticals, presents a genuine cause for concern regarding human health[271]. Again, this supports the recommendation that supplements should only be taken when specifically recommended by an appropriately qualified medical expert.

Along similar lines, and introducing another problem that has been associated with calcium supplements, a recent study in the US reported that 90% of calcium supplements were contaminated with unacceptably high concentrations of lead[272]. The issue of supplement contamination is not limited to mineral tablets alone.

A recent Canadian study of omega-3 supplements reported low-level contamination by pollutants in those manufactured from salmon, tuna and sea-herring[273], although the levels were lower than would be found in fresh fish. The recommendation from this study was to use supplements manufactured from small, oily fish, such as sardines and mackerel. Omega-3 supplements could be one of the only supplements really beneficial to the majority of people (or rather those who do not obtain sufficient omega-3 fats from other sources). Of particular note, omega-3 fats are processed to a consistently high standard, and any pollutants present are typically found to be in lower concentrations than those from fresh fish sources.

* * * * * * *

Regulatory control and enforcement of legislation regarding supplements is a huge problem. Supplements are not seen as medicines, and as such are not regulated or controlled as medicines. Supplements require no evidence *whatsoever* to demonstrate effectiveness, and there is scant research available on their efficacy and even their side-effects. Even worse, the manufacturers typically fund the little evidence that does exist, and any research funded by a manufacturer is more likely to demonstrate effectiveness than an independent study. But then, so few researchers want to spend their time investigating supplements anyway, especially as every few months new pills and potions come onto the market, or the nutrient compositions of existing brands change, all of which makes the research out of date and redundant anyway. A recent study[274], has highlighted some of these issues, including contamination, the lack of public awareness, and the need for improved quality control.

A failure to advertise the potential harm caused by nutritional supplements can have severe repercussions. One recent report[275] detailed two patients who suffered heart attacks after consuming unusually high quantities of potassium. In individuals with normal kidney function a potassium overdose is highly unlikely, but the inclusion of potassium in supplements and salt substitutes provides individuals with the chance to overdose, and many people are unlikely to be aware of this. The consequences of potassium overdose include multiple organ failure, muscular weakness, cardiac abnormalities and paralysis[275]. Again, although very unusual it does happen, and it only happens due to assumptions about supplements and health, and a lack of clear information from healthcare professionals.

Some weight-loss supplements have been found to cause significant liver injury[276], including Hydroxycut[277], Herbalife(R)[278], tea extracts and products containing usnic acid and high concentrations of vitamin A[279,280]. Other weight-loss supplements have been associated with severe cardiovascular incidents, and even death[281]. Hydroxycut and Herbalife(R) weight-loss formulas are still widely available, although the formulations have been altered following awareness of the liver injury cases. Other supplements reported to be used for weight-loss but found to cause harm include chromium, tea extract and tea root extract, yohimbine, ephedra (*Ma huang*), Garcinia cambogia extract, Hoodia gordoni and Dong quai[277]. It should be added that tea itself is typically quite healthy, but taking a very concentrated form or extract is not how tea is naturally consumed, and in some cases this can lead to adverse effects.

Health is about balance in all aspects of our personal physiology – whenever something is altered beyond its natural set-point, so the body reacts to bring everything back into balance. The body can increase metabolism or slow it down, it can heat itself up or promote heat loss, can increase water retention or reduce it. The key is that the body strives to maintain its state of balance – free from extremes of anything. Really then, health is about ensuring we obtain enough of what we need, and avoid generating imbalances by overloading it with high concentrations of particular substances. We need just enough, and too much of anything can be just as bad as not enough. The chances are, and as harsh to our intellects as it may sound, our bodies are probably far better at maintaining balance without us complicating the processes by overloading ourselves with supplements.

A thorough review of the literature[334] concluded that health claims associated with Ginkgo biloba lacked evidence, and neither safety nor efficacy could be guaranteed. The investigators reported that 25 of 29 Ginkgo biloba supplements tested did not contain the required minimum concentration of extract, and in most there were significant discrepancies between what was contained in the supplement and what was listed on the label. A safe maximum dosage could not be established due to a lack of available research[334].

It remains the case that all supplements are manufactured and marketed without the requirement for thorough, rigorous and long-term evidence of safety and effectiveness. That people are willing to consume such supplements, without any objective evidence they work, implies it must follow effective marketing or personal recommendations. However, that lack of evidence means it is an act of faith, belief, assumption and a desire for them to work, and nothing more. That there is such variable quality amongst supplements and a lack of evidence, even of basic safety, indicates consumers need to be far more demanding than they currently are, and this is a matter requiring the support of effective regulatory bodies.

* * * * * * *

Whilst some studies have investigated the effects of certain supplements on cancer prevention[282,283,334,336] there is insufficient evidence of direct effects of novel supplements and cancer prevention or treatment. Similarly, a recent systematic review[284] found there was no evidence to either support or refute the use of anti-oxidant supplements amongst patients with liver disease. Another review assessed various different Chinese herbal formulas used to protect the liver[285], and reported that studies were typically of a poor standard, with little regard for adverse effects or controlling bias. The investigators reported that, because so many ingredients were contained within each of the Chinese herbal formulas, it was not possible to determine which substances were meant to be the active ingredients. The review concluded that the absence of supporting evidence of those Chinese herbal medicines, demonstrated the need to stop prescribing them, particularly considering a lack of reporting on adverse effects[285].

Mineral supplements can prevent absorption of anti-oxidants, including vitamins C and E[286]. Further, supplemental vitamin C has been used in some studies to deliberately increase oxidative stress[286].

Importantly, the minerals within multivitamin/mineral supplements have been demonstrated to inhibit the absorption of anti-oxidant vitamins[286] in a way that cannot happen in natural foods. This is because in a tablet or pill there are minerals together with water-soluble and fat-soluble vitamins, whereas in real foods the nutrients are within plant or animal matter and are processed more effectively for absorption.

Despite the intake of supplements amongst the general public being very high[287], a recent study of Olympic athletes[288] reported that total consumption of nutritional supplements has been decreasing. Considering that high doses of anti-oxidants can potentially interfere with normal anti-oxidant pathways, and can in some cases cause more harm, this is a promising development. Some supplements can provide benefits, but it is unusual for this to be the case in individuals already consuming a healthy diet. Unfortunately it is beyond the scope of this book to discuss many individual supplements specifically, but creatine and caffeine have shown promise for certain athlete groups. The general consumption of multivitamins/minerals or herbal products is not sufficiently supported, and in some cases is contra-indicated entirely.

* * * * * * *

Herbal extracts are the basis for many modern medicines. The task of pharmaceuticals companies has been to find the active ingredients within a medicinal plant, extract it and then test it. Those who dislike or distrust the pharmaceuticals industry might favour many commercially available, 'natural' remedies, but favouring an inadequately regulated industry over an established, tested one is not logically the better alternative. Herbal remedies contain more of the plant than simply the active ingredient, and as plants contain various substances there to protect them from being eaten, a plant extract will likely contain poisons as well as medicinal components. These potentially harmful substances are typically fine when the plant is eaten as a food, but when it is made into an extract the concentrations of both beneficial and harmful ingredients can increase dramatically. The lack of regulation means it is likely that 'natural' plant-based remedies can be more harmful than commonly available pharmaceuticals.

In a book on *Our Natural Diet* it might be assumed this is some sort of hypocrisy, but the reality is that both pharmaceuticals and natural remedies are based upon plant extracts. The pharmaceuticals industry invests millions on funding researchers to find the active, medicinal properties of a plant, after which the manufacturer must jump through hoops to establish safety, including reporting of side effects which have to be included on labelling and information sheets. The results of those studies are then published and available, and passed over to medical establishments for judgements to be made on whether or not they will be made available to patients. This is not a perfect system, and there are gaps, deliberate deceptions, and biased research papers published. However, natural remedies *have no regulations whatsoever* regarding effectiveness in treating medical conditions, and often no labelling regarding side effects. The debates regarding the use of pharmaceuticals are beyond the scope of a book on diet, but Ben Goldacre introduces many salient points in his book *Bad Science*.

The executive summary is that pharmaceuticals, supplements and herbal remedies are far from perfect, but to accept that so-called natural or herbal remedies are better, just because the name sounds right, can be a disastrous assumption. The author of a recent review of supplements for anxiety-related disorders, stated that even though some herbal remedies do produce positive results, identifying the active ingredients can be difficult, with consumers exposed to ineffective and possibly harmful substances[289]. Natural yes, but whether or not the balance tips towards the healthful or harmful is typically not known even by the manufacturers, and whether or not the end product can be indicated for use is most often a mystery. Further, the above refers to herbal remedies for anxiety disorders, a few of which do have reasonable support for their efficacy, but the lack of regulation and knowledge of side-effects makes it impossible to recommend them at present.

Some supplements do confer indisputable benefits to those individuals who genuinely need them, but even at best their role is to supplement a deficient diet, not to improve an already adequate one, and almost never to treat illness. In some cases, supplements have been shown to be cost-effective and useful in promoting the health status of malnourished patients[290]. However, any greater claims than this are typically not well researched, and are the claims of individuals in marketing roles, not medical researchers.

Toxins

*"If you are young and you drink a great deal it will spoil
your health, slow your mind, make you fat
– in other words, turn you into an adult."*

- P. J. O'Rourke

The intention with this chapter was to give a general overview of what is meant by the term 'toxins', and then go into some specific examples and details. That so much has been written is really reflective of the volume of misinformation and pseudoscience relating to the topic. So, although it was intended that all readers would enjoy this whole chapter, some will probably want to read a little and then skip through, whilst others more keen to see 'how deep the rabbit hole goes' might be more interested in some of the specific chemicals mentioned. In any case, this chapter aims to offer something for everyone, rather than everything for only the few.

The difficulty we have is that although there undoubtedly *are* toxins, or rather substances that have toxic effects, the use of 'toxins' as an umbrella term, referring to any non-specific thing we might not want, has made most of the debate entirely meaningless and nonsensical.

During the academic year in which this book was written (2010-11), at the college where I work not a single student in their final year project viva included the term 'toxin', and this was taken as a sign of progress. Either the students had listened carefully to their instructions regarding this, or else the warnings from students assessed in previous years had been passed down. An example would help here. During the assessments the previous year, a student was describing breathing exercises commonly used in a type of yoga, and tried to explain that these breathing exercises removed toxins. On the assessment panel sat a physiologist (self), a biochemist and neuroscientist, and an external examiner with a background in nutrition and physiology. From the students' first year we had all warned them against the non-specific use of the term toxins.

When we challenged the student to describe which toxins she meant, specifically, she was unable to say, so kept repeating the word 'toxins', hoping that would help the penny to drop and we would suddenly know what she meant. When she later resubmitted her dissertation, she changed the word toxin to carbon dioxide. So, the benefit of her breathing exercises, according to her, was that they helped remove carbon dioxide from the body. But the exercises involved deep breathing, meaning that more oxygen was taken in, which in itself could increase ROS production, and the only reason more carbon dioxide would leave would be if more were generated by the cells.

Further, if that were actually happening, the breathing exercises would be creating more of these *toxins* for the body to remove. In other words, more toxins could only be removed from the body if more were created. The body always works to maintain balance of all these things, so the idea that breathing deeply will somehow create benefits above breathing as the body is content to breathe is an unfounded assumption; it also seems to be logically wrong. However, there is insufficient scope here to drag breathing exercises through the wringer entirely. There is a place for them, but that place has more to do with physical therapy and meditation, and all the benefits they confer to physical and mental well-being. There is no need to try and add to that with woolly and factually incorrect pseudoscience.

What is perhaps most telling is that, although some research scientists qualify as *toxicologists* there is no such thing as a *detoxicologist*. The problem is that 'detox' is also a meaningless term unless it is applied specifically. Oxidative stress can be caused from by-products of metabolism, but as has been discussed the same substances can act as either anti-oxidants or pro-oxidants, and both roles are essential for normal health. We can describe oxygen, nitrogen, water and all foods as toxins, because they all have the capacity to harm the body, but as they are all essential and we cannot live without them it seems ridiculous to entertain the idea. So, with most 'toxins' being by-products of normal breathing and metabolism, we have to accept that whilst almost 100% of these are a benefit, the tiny excess fraction that can cause harm is all that requires attention. We do not need to stop breathing, eating or moving to 'detoxify', because the body is already highly efficient at neutralising the miniscule amounts with the potential for harm.

We can bolster our protective systems by consuming plenty of fruits and vegetables and reducing stressors in our daily life, but for the greatest 'toxin' contributors to our bodies we absolutely cannot 'detoxify' in any meaningful way. We breathe, we urinate and we defecate. If anyone wishes to regard those as detoxification then so be it, and I deny nobody the privilege. Further, because the 'toxic' reactions take place at a rate of millions of reactions a second, and are neutralised just as quickly, it is equally meaningless to suppose that these 'toxins' build up, because they do not. People can have a good balance between anti-oxidant and pro-oxidant processes, which will have benefits for whole body health, but this is through ensuring a sufficient intake of fruits and vegetables, engaging in plenty of physical activity, and striving to reduce stress in daily life.

So, this accounts for almost 100% of all toxins we are exposed to, and although detoxification is meaningless in this sense, there is justification in maintaining a healthy, oxidant balance that lends itself to healthy blood vessels and healthy cells, tissues and organs. This is accomplished through the management of diet and lifestyle factors. If we can accept this, then it is appropriate to discuss other toxins.

* * * * * * *

We do expose ourselves to substances that have toxic effects on the body, in addition to the natural and naturally neutralised by-products of breathing and metabolism. These are specific chemicals, and so can be referred to either by their name, or the cells, tissues or organs upon which they might have their harmful effect. For example, alcohol is a neurotoxin, meaning that it can damage nerve cells. It is also a hepatotoxin, meaning it can damage liver cells. Some metal contaminants in foods can be nephrotoxins, meaning they can harm the kidneys. So, the three main target areas are the nerve and brain cells (neurotoxins), the liver (hepatotoxins) and kidneys (nephrotoxins). There are other specific effects of certain chemicals; as discussed in the chapter on supplements, calcium can directly damage blood vessel walls, although that we need calcium makes it difficult for us to describe calcium as a toxin. We could say that some calcium supplements have been found to contain a metal toxin – lead – because lead can cause harm, but why not be specific and call it lead rather than be non-specific and refer to it only as a toxin? We know where we are with lead; we can look at research to find its specific effects, how those effects are limited and how the tissues repair. The bottom line will of course be to stop taking supplements containing lead, and that is all the 'detox' required.

Hence, there is a general dislike from many scientists of this umbrella term of toxins, which does not really mean anything unless we are describing a specific toxic effect of a specific substance. We can talk about the harmful effects of high concentrations of calcium, but we cannot really describe it as a toxin in its own right, nor can we 'detoxify' ourselves of calcium, particularly if we enjoy living. Lead is a toxin in the right sense, but why not just be specific? Presumably, people talk about toxins in general because they do not know exactly which chemicals they are referring to, and if they did we would probably find they are actually talking about normal, natural substances, which generate normal, natural responses within the body.

The issue of a given substance being potentially both essential *and* toxic is further complicated by the fact some substances only have harmful consequences in certain individuals, such as those with specific organ defects. Glucose becomes harmful in high concentrations, but the body's natural homeostatic mechanisms are effective in preventing this from occurring. So, for the majority of people glucose is not a toxin. However, this is not necessarily the case in diabetics, because their homeostatic mechanisms are inadequate to maintain glucose levels within those healthy limits. The consequences of this can include damage to cells of the immune system, nerve cells, the eyes and kidneys[291].

Preventing or limiting the effects of glucose cannot be managed by any 'detox' strategy, but simply comes down to managing carbohydrate intake and promoting a healthy oxidant status, and – unsurprisingly – including plenty of fruits and vegetables in the diet. In some cases diabetics will have to take insulin or similar, but this is a natural substance and difficult to regard as a 'detoxifying' chemical. Glucose is one of the main energy sources for the body, and is the primary energy source for the brain, so it is fairly clear this cannot and should not be avoided (unless a ketogenic diet is recommended on a specific, individual basis).

Some toxins are not essential for normal daily living, but might be a by-product of a drug taken to treat a specific condition[292]. The consequences of drug-induced kidney damage can be severe, but people would not willingly expose themselves to this and the benefit-to-cost ratio would have to indicate that the risks were worth it. Again, dietary and lifestyle management should promote kidney protection, and any prescribed drugs should not be taken above recommended dosages or for any longer than required.

Kidney damage can also be caused by faults within the cells themselves[293], with the damage being oxidative stress, which should be protected against through diet and lifestyle factors. There is a clear trend here. Prior to this chapter the word toxin was not used at all in this book, because it was appropriate and easy enough to refer to specific chemicals each time. Within this chapter, even with the more generic use of 'toxins', it is still clear that protection comes from normal dietary and lifestyle management.

The message really is that we need to be far more sceptical of the generic, non-specific and deliberately confusing use of the terms toxins and detox. The following questions should follow naturally when the subject of toxins or detox arises: which toxins specifically, what do they do, and how is this normally prevented, managed or treated? If we are deliberately putting a harmful substance into ourselves, we need to stop doing so. How hard can it be?

* * * * * * *

The liver is the main organ involved in dealing with waste products, drugs, environmental chemicals, and generally anything the body needs to have processed in some way, so as to reduce the harm it can cause before it is removed from the body. Because the liver has to be exposed to these substances before they can be removed, the cells of the liver are at risk of damage themselves[294]. Ensuring the liver can recover from exposures to harmful substances requires a healthy diet. However, the most important step is to limit exposure to potentially harmful chemicals in the first place, rather than willingly cause damage and try and fix everything afterwards.

The liver processes substances produced naturally within the body, in addition to those that reach the blood from the air, foods and drink. Airborne pollutants, chemical preservatives in foods, and pharmaceuticals – amongst other sources of potentially harmful substances – will sooner or later pass through the liver. The best protection is certainly not 'detox', whatever that means, but avoidance or limiting of exposure in the first place. If exposure does occur, then it is best to ensure it is minimal and short-term, with the next step being to promote recovery. Minimising exposure from foods can be managed by eating a variety of foods, as single exposures to harmful substances are typically insufficient to cause irreversible harm (high doses of radiation perhaps being an exception, as could be some drugs, although not the sorts commercially available).

* * * * * * *

Usually, damage from nutritional toxins, such as alcohol, occur through ingestion of very high amounts (i.e. binge drinking), or through long-term high exposures (alcoholism). Alcohol itself can harm nerve cells (brain and nervous system) and liver cells. Alcoholism can lead to problems with liver function and nerves involved in sense, movement and signalling to organs (peripheral neuropathies)[295]. Short-term exposure to high concentrations of ethanol, as occurs during binge drinking, can lead to tremors, hallucinations, seizures, and fluctuations in alertness and agitation. Long term, the damage to nerve cells can contribute to serious disorders, including dementia[296]. Ethanol intake is also associated with impaired learning and memory deficiencies. There are also changes in the structural and fluid components of the brain, including a loss of cells, prevention of cell growth and interference in normal signalling pathways[296].

The protective effects of red wine are due largely to the phytochemicals from the grapes, or else the preferable lifestyles of people who drink wine rather than other types of alcohol. Hence, in this sense it is more appropriate to recommend a healthy lifestyle and a diet rich in phytochemicals, rather than to increase wine intake. However, a low intake of alcohol has been shown to be beneficial to blood vessels, and this is something related to ethanol itself and not the phytochemical content of certain drinks. So, low intakes of alcohol do appear to be genuinely beneficial in some regards, although these benefits are no different to the benefits of a healthy lifestyle and diet anyway.

Binge drinking during adolescence can cause real problems to the developing brain, affecting hormone levels and promoting risks of behavioural problems. Drinking during pregnancy exposes the foetus to alcohol, as this passes from the mother into the foetal circulation. Foetal Alcohol Syndrome (FAS) is the leading cause of non-genetic mental disability, although its prevalence is under-reported[297]. Foetal exposure to ethanol increases the risk of central nervous system defects, growth deficiencies, facial abnormalities, and anomalies of the heart, skeleton, genitals, skin, and muscles. Specific effects can include mental retardation, poor coordination, hyperactivity and other behavioural problems, and muscle contraction problems. Some of these consequences of ethanol exposure can be long lasting, and persist into adulthood, and unfortunately there is a risk even with low intakes[297].

We can make a conscious decision to drink less, less often, or to avoid it entirely. No pill, breathing exercise or other alternative 'detox' therapy can remove ethanol or damaged cells from the liver. A low energy 'detox' diet will likely cause even more problems, because the protection and regeneration of harmed liver cells requires plenty of anti-oxidants, fats, cholesterol and proteins. So, ethanol and other such harmful chemicals do not build-up in the body, but their presence before they are eliminated can cause damage. Because the liver is so exposed to these substances, it has become incredibly effective at removing and regenerating cells. Hence, an occasional alcoholic drink may cause transient damage, but the cells will quickly repair themselves. An extended exposure (alcoholism) or very high single exposures (binge-drinking) present a risk because the cells might not regenerate before the next exposure, facilitating serious liver damage.

* * * * * * *

There are certainly some environmental toxins, which are not a naturally occurring constituent of foods or the air, but which can be taken up into plants, into the animals that eat plants, into water sources, or released into the air directly from industry. We can be specific, so as not to fall victim to the generic use of the term we are striving to avoid (although to do so perhaps shows why it can be preferable to using the long-winded names of these materials).

MIBK (methyl isobutyl ketone, if you prefer) is an important industrial chemical that can be found in rubbing alcohol, paints, varnishes, as a solvent in protective coatings, in dry-cleaning preparations and various other substances[298]. The people most at risk will work directly with this chemical, and it can cause problems if exposed to the skin, eyes, or through inhalation. Once in the bloodstream MIBK is distributed around the body, and has been shown to affect the kidneys and livers of rodents, increasing risk of tumours[298]. Limiting exposure would be through avoiding work that involves manufacturing MIBK-containing products, and ensuring that any contact with skin or eyes is avoided. Again, there is no 'detox', but rather a limiting of exposure in the first place.

Some heavy metals can occur in agricultural soils, and the concentrations will vary depending upon how the land is used and which chemicals the soil is exposed to. Excessive chemical fertilizers and organic manures can lead to an increase in the concentrations of heavy metals within crops grown in such soil[299]. Because these metals, such as zinc and copper, are essential, it is difficult to consider them as being a toxin, although they can certainly cause serious harm to blood vessels, cells and organs when in excess[300,299].

Some chemicals that are taken up from soil into plants are not required at all, such as arsenic[299,301] and cadmium[299,302]. The concentrations vary from plant species to species, and favouring vegetables grown on organic land, or home-grown, is preferable to avoid exposure. When that is not possible, trying to include a wide variety of vegetables from various locations will help limit excessive intakes of any one particular metal.

Acrylamide (ACR) is a chemical used in water and wastewater management, and is formed during high-temperature processing of some potato- and grain-based products[303]. ACR can be neurotoxic and cause muscle weakness, problems with movement, balance and speech, and affect mental status. Regulations are required to ensure that ACR produced within foods is monitored and kept within safe limits, although potato and cereal grains likely to have been exposed to high temperatures during processing could be avoided.

There is an almost overwhelming volume of research available regarding the risks and benefits of nitrates and nitrites. We are exposed to these chemicals in tap water, their uptake from the soil into vegetables, and as chemical preservatives in foods. These substances are also produced naturally within the body. A whole chapter could easily be dedicated to this issue (and almost was). The summary is that nitrates and nitrites produced naturally within the body are an important element of human health, and although harmful in high quantities we cannot be without them if we wish to be healthy. However, high quantities of nitrates and nitrites have been associated with various types of cancer, including stomach cancer.

Regulations are in place to ensure that tap water concentrations are maintained within safe limits, although anyone concerned can opt for mineral water, steam-distilled water or having a reverse-osmosis water filter fitted beneath their sink. Because fruits and vegetables are protective against damage, the benefits of consuming these far outweigh the costs. It would be worthwhile avoiding intake of foods that have nitrates or nitrites *added* to them, such as many preserved meats.

In some cases, it is not the food itself that contains the harmful substances in nature, but rather the chemicals can leach into the food during or after processing. Canned food can contain BADGE (2,2-bis(4-hydroxyphenyl)propane bis(2,3-epoxypropyl) ether – to give it its full title, which is almost enough to make me prefer the term 'toxin'). This is a chemical used in the manufacture of the lacquers for coating the inside of food and drinks cans. BADGE has been shown to move from the coatings of cans and into the foods, but in some cases the concentrations are far too low to present a health concern, whilst in others they are not detected in the foods at all[304]. However, consuming a lot of canned foods regularly would increase total exposure[305].

The most appropriate recommendation is to prefer fresh foods over canned, and opt for drinks from glass bottles. Considering the actual risk to health is so minimal, this recommendation is taking matters further than they really need to go. Again, we are limiting exposure to 'toxins' rather than attempting to detoxify afterwards, because all *detox* can be is the natural elimination of these substances, and the prevention, management and treatment of harm through bolstering anti-oxidant defences in a natural manner. Tap water can become contaminated with heavy metals, which can subsequently lead to nerve damage[306], however exposure requires the contaminants to reach drinking water and this is highly unusual. In regions where it is known that drinking water is contaminated, it would be appropriate to consume bottled water instead, but, as stated elsewhere, there are very few water supplies contaminated sufficiently to pose real concerns for human health.

Another environmental toxin is MVK (methyvinyl ketone), which is used in the production of pesticides, perfumes, plastics, resins, and laboratory-synthesised steroid hormones, vitamin A and anti-coagulants[307]. Exposure of rats to MVK leads to severe damage to the upper respiratory tract, affecting body weight, lung weight and leading to death following a single high exposure. A longer-term study suggested damage to the testes of males, and to the kidneys and livers of the rodents tested[307]. It is difficult to think of any recommendation other than limiting exposure to vapour in the manufacture of substances containing MVK.

Methamphetamine is a psychostimulant and often taken

recreationally. However, it has also been prescribed as a treatment for narcolepsy and ADHD. Methamphetamine is also a potent neurotoxin, and can be used in animals to develop Parkinson's disease, so as to permit researchers to investigate treatments for the condition[308]. General anaesthetics have also been found to have neurotoxic effects, with the potential to cause long-term harm to the brain. The underlying mechanisms appear to be related to oxidative stress[309], supporting a case for ensuring oxidant balance is maintained

* * * * * * *

One of the most common mechanisms by which a toxin damages the cells of the body is through oxidative and nitrosative stress. Despite a fair amount of this book including descriptions and recommendations of anti-oxidant and pro-oxidant processes, and how certain nutrients can be involved in these, it is important to state that researchers do not have the technology available to fully understand all the underlying mechanisms and interactions. The research currently available tends to use markers, or signals, of oxidative and nitrosative damage, and of the protection offered by anti-oxidants, but these are all indirect measures[310].

Considerable scepticism should be directed at anyone making strong claims about generic toxins and *detoxification*. The notion that a non-researcher knows about some system, strategy, exercise, supplement or diet that detoxifies is a nonsense. Which toxin(s)? What harm do they do? Are there benefits from these substances? How does the body usually manage them, both normally and when in excess? How does this system/strategy/exercise/supplement/diet interact with this particular substance to ensure only benefits are

199

derived, with normal anti-oxidant/pro-oxidant systems not being interfered with?

Considering our lack of understanding of anti-oxidant/pro-oxidant signalling within cells, and the lack of accurate reporting on these issues in the media, a non-researcher in this field will know so much less than the active scientists investigating the topic. In any case, all of the evidence currently available demonstrates it is far more complicated and substance-specific than is typically reported in the press. Further, all the evidence demonstrates the most appropriate approach is to avoid or limit exposure to environmental toxins, and to bolster our natural anti-oxidant/pro-oxidative systems through a diet rich in a variety of fruits and vegetables, omega-3 fats, plenty of physical activity, and a reduction in daily stress. This might not seem particularly exciting, dynamic, fashionable or sexy, but it is sensible, logical and supported by the considerable weight of available scientific evidence.

> *"The body is a big sagacity, a plurality with one sense,*
> *a war and a peace, a flock and a shepherd."*
>
> **- Friedrich Nietzsche**

Weight Management

*"If nature had intended our skeletons to be visible
it would have put them on the outside of our bodies."*

- Elmer Rice

Considering that entire books are dedicated to weight-loss specifically, this chapter is fairly brief as an attempt to consolidate the essential points into a justly appropriate volume of text. Anyone with a reasonable understanding of nutrition and metabolism will appreciate that weight management is about the balance of energy taken in and energy used up. If someone expends more energy than they ingest (negative energy balance), they will lose weight, whereas if they consume more energy than they use (positive energy balance) they will gain weight. Simple?

Well, the science of weight loss is incredibly straightforward in principle, at least in terms of the physiology of how to lose weight. It is perhaps deliberately over-complicated for the sake of selling a product, or convincing people of a system, but this is not justified by the actual science of dieting – however sciencey it might be made to seem. Perhaps the other side is that when people do not have success with a particular approach, after a while there might be a belief the system(s) failed because the authors overlooked some important aspect of science, and so a new system based upon a deeper understanding of dieting is required. However, after decades of seeing different dieting books and systems come and go, it seems that more recent books do not tend to demonstrate a deeper understanding of our biology, but rather a *different* understanding of it. However, regardless of the basis for a particular diet, the chances are it will fall short because it fails to support a long-term energy deficit. This is typically due to the restrictions in what can be eaten leading to deficiencies in key nutrients, which leads to either cravings or other negative effects. Whatever the underlying shortcomings of the diet, ultimately it means the dieter is unable to maintain the diet long-term. Reducing energy-intake – however that is achieved – will cause feelings of hunger, and over an extended period of time that will have all sorts of psychological repercussions.

Cravings and fatigue are less likely on a nutrient-dense diet. Having stated that *physiologically* dieting is very straightforward, it is equally true that *psychologically* dieting can be incredibly stressful, onerous and challenging (with rewards often not seen soon enough to compensate and promote motivation). Behavioural change strategies are developed and promoted to support people through long-term weight loss programmes, but if the actual diet is inadequate then people will work too hard – and suffer too much – for what is unlikely to be long-term success. Committing to be healthy – to prioritise and focus upon a healthy diet and active lifestyle – is the most important yet overlooked first step.

If someone is committed to being healthy, they will tend to eat healthier foods, which happen to be relatively low in energy compared with processed and convenience foods, but very high in good quality nutrients. A commitment to health will also tend to make people want to increase their daily physical activity levels, promoting the energy deficit and permitting greater and longer-lasting weight loss than can be obtained through dieting alone. In short, by maximising intake of a very high-quality, nutrient-dense diet, it is far harder to consume too much energy, and much easier to avoid cravings.

* * * * * * *

Writing as a physiologist, the psychological aspects of dieting are by far the most important, because the motivation, desire, willingness and commitment are the real yet overlooked requirements for long-term weight-loss. It does sound obvious, but somehow the physiology of weight-loss seems to be the main focus of diets: calorie-counting, nutrient-percentages, multiple dietary phases, tests, and so on.

Physiologically all we can really do is make the dieting process easier by promoting sufficient nutrient intake and supporting an overall energy-deficit. Hence, a maximally healthy diet is more likely to be maintained and is more effective for long-term weight management, because it limits the body's cravings for the neglected nutrients. So, there is a limit to the advice that can be given in this regard: eat a healthy diet, rich in all the key foods described in this book, and prioritise a physically-active lifestyle. Once someone has committed to their health and weight-loss, there is very little need for dietary 'instruction', because people tend to eat healthier by choice and want to expend more energy on a daily basis.

The psychological factors overrule everything else, and a diet will succeed or fail based upon those – how 'good' the diet is in terms of its incorporated foods and weight-loss strategies only makes the weight-loss process easier or harder, but it is the psychological determination and commitment that determines whether or not the person reaches their goal. Everything in between tends to be hard work, and a sub-standard diet is more likely to cause someone to throw in the towel before he or she reaches their target bodyweight or body composition. In this sense, it seems that typical diets are not effective because they attempt to force weight loss through abrupt changes, and so are antagonistic to our sense of comfort, ease and satisfaction. Conversely, a healthy diet – which is not in itself designed to promote weight loss – becomes the more effective simply because it should be more comfortable, satisfying and easy to maintain for life. All that needs to be influenced is the total amount of energy going in, and the total amount of physical activity to support and promote weight-loss.

Perhaps the reason for 'fad' diets is that people can commit to a few weeks, or even a couple of months without too much trouble, but then once the motivation runs out the next diet along facilitates the new impetus. In all cases, long-term success comes from a healthy diet, not a short-term fad diet with limits in important nutrients. But there does seem to be so much 'science' surrounding dieting, and that needs to be discussed, even if purely to demonstrate why weight-loss should not be based upon calorie-counting or other traditional and sciencey strategies.

* * * * * * *

One thing that complicates the fairly straightforward physiology of it all is in how we calculate energy intake, which is not at all accurate, or even really meaningful. The whole matter of understanding energy intake is further complicated by fluctuations in normal metabolic processes, which vary between and within individuals, and which can be influenced by long-term overweightness/obesity. When we attempt to become scientific about weight loss we actually see how the 'science' commonly used as a tool is in fact a misleading hindrance.

To begin with, if I, as a physiologist, wish to measure someone's metabolism, I can invite them into my lab and have them breathe into a unit that records the air they expire. This can be done at rest or during exercise, and the sampled air will give me information about total energy being used, and the proportions of carbohydrates, fats and proteins providing the fuels. This gives a snapshot of what the person's metabolism is like at that time of day, and will be affected by recent meals, recent physical activity, other stresses, how much sleep they had, the temperature and various other factors.

A more appropriate test might be a 24-hour stint in a metabolic chamber, in which the same measures can be taken but whilst the individual moves around in a room, spends a few minutes on a treadmill or bike, sleeps for a while, and so on. This is a 24-hour record, so more realistic as a representation of the truth than a few minutes, but it is at best only a single day – and a day spent in an enclosed space at that. Actual metabolism will still differ according to dietary and lifestyle factors, so even the most sophisticated scientific measures are only an indication. Any significant changes in diet, lifestyle, stress or fitness will have marked effects on metabolism and which foods provide however much energy.

On this basis it should be clear that any online metabolic rate calculators, or printed calculations that use information such as body weight, height, percentage body fat, resting heart rate and so on – however sophisticated the equations can be – are really only very crude estimates, and should not be viewed as particularly accurate on an individual level. So, energy used on a daily basis is highly variable and cannot be measured in a truly meaningful, accurate way – the best we can manage is a reasonable indication, about which will be some considerable fluctuations. How about the other side of the equation – calculating energy intake?

Well, if someone is ingesting food and drink, they are taking sources of energy into the body. Again, there are those who would like to dictate to others that – once their resting metabolic rate has been calculated – someone's weight can be increased, decreased or kept in balance by ensuring energy intake is greater, lower, or equivalent to metabolic rate, respectively. Considering that metabolic rate is only ever crudely estimated, it is reasonable to assume that matching energy intake with energy losses (metabolic rate) in this way is open to some error. The reality, however, is that it is far far more farcical than this. Do individuals who recommend this approach, for example, assume that those they are advising excrete faeces and urine with a zero energy content? This would be energy lost that is not taken into account when measuring metabolism, and as waste from the gut includes foods not absorbed into the blood, much cannot be counted as 'energy in', if we are being entirely accurate.

How much energy is contained within a meal will have an effect on the rate the food leaves the stomach (gastric emptying), which will influence how much is absorbed into the blood and how much passes out of the body unabsorbed[311,312]. In fact, gastric emptying will be affected by many disease states, such as diabetes, ulcers, cancers and post-surgery. Further, it will be influenced by hormone levels, emotional state, medication, how much of the meal is solid and how much is liquid and the relative amounts of carbohydrates, fats and proteins[311]. The energy and nutrient content of a breakfast will affect the gastric emptying of lunch, and have effects on subsequent food intake and satiety[313].

This is all further obscured by the variability between individuals consuming the same meals, and that energy is produced within the gut through interactions between foods and bacteria, which contribute to overall energy but are difficult to estimate[314]. The total energy content of a meal will affect how the gut bacteria interact with the foods, how much of those foods is absorbed and how much is excreted[315].

There is a relationship between the amount of fat in a meal

and the amount of fat in the faeces, but it is a weak relationship, which makes accurate calculations of the fat contribution to total energy impossible[314]. How much protein, fat and carbohydrate are excreted in faeces will depend upon the amount and type of fibre in a meal, again complicating any estimates of total energy content[316]. The effects of fibre on the body are still poorly understood, and we have an insufficient knowledge of which types of fibre are metabolised into energy, which react with bacteria to promote energy, and which promote the removal of nutrients from the gut and reduce energy available for absorption[316].

* * * * * * *

Perhaps the most obvious problem with attempting to use a 'scientific' approach to manipulating energy balance relates to the way in which energy is calculated, or more specifically what the numbers actually refer to. When measuring metabolic energy the numbers given are in either kilocalories or kilojoules. Similarly, food labels include an energy content with the same units – either calories (referring to kilocalories, 'kcals') or kilojoules. Does this mean that if ten 'food label' calories of carbohydrate were absorbed from a food into the blood, it would provide ten calories of energy that could be measured via assessments of metabolic rate?

Well, if a meal contains 500 kilocalories, for example, the one thing we know for sure is that 500 kcals will not be entering the blood. Interactions between that meal and gut bacteria will generate more energy, whilst the fibres within the meal and other bacteria will ensure some of that energy is excreted without being absorbed. What makes the notion of finding a balance even more ridiculous is that the calories and joules from a meal do not relate to metabolic processes. That an apple has 50 kcals and a chocolate bar has 250 kcals absolutely does not mean that the chocolate bar provides five-times more energy than an apple. The problem here comes down to the process of *bomb calorimetry*.

In order to calculate the energy content of a food, that food can be placed into a sealed container and combusted, using a piece of apparatus known as a bomb calorimeter. These are not really used for this purpose anymore, as manufacturers use fairly old data based on a set energy content of fat (about 9-kcals per gram), carbohydrate (about 4-kcals per gram), and protein (about 4-kcals per gram). So, one problem is that as there are so many interactions between these nutrients during processing, cooking and digestion, we do not know how much of the original energy content is actually available for absorption. The biggest problem, however, is that the body does not combust foods like a bomb calorimeter, but instead breaks foods down through chemical processing and mechanical breakdown, from the moment the food enters the mouth to the point that the derivative of the original substance is converted into chemical energy and used.

The problem is even further complicated by hormonal actions that are dependent upon body fat stores. Hormonal factors affect appetite and whether or not food is stored as fat[317], thereby complicating the issue of whether or not an absorbed amount of food provides a predictable amount of energy. This is particularly the case for people who have been overweight for a long time, who may have a less efficient sense of when their appetite is sated as a result, and may be more likely to store fat than someone who is lean, as has been found in individuals who produce a faulty type of the hormone leptin. Some people do like to become very absorbed with the science of nutrition, but the science has its limits, particularly when attempting to exploit the science for the needs of an individual.

Calculating food calories is highly inaccurate on every conceivable level, and calculating metabolic rate as a means to know energy usage is so crude as to be virtually meaningless anyway. The best way for an individual to manage or manipulate their energy balance is to keep a check on their lifestyle and what they are eating, how much, when, and what their body weight is. If someone has maintained their weight for a few months, then it is a fair assumption they are in a state of energy balance.

Losing weight requires eating less, and/or doing more exercise. Long-term, the most effective means of weight-loss is a combination of diet and exercise, which has been shown to be more effective and sustainable than diet restriction alone. In short, the most scientifically accurate, useful and meaningful approach is to focus on the individual and their current dietary and lifestyle habits, and to manipulate that rather than dictate calorie requirements.

People are better at subconsciously managing energy intake to ensure consistency than might be assumed. One study[318] has shown that when people consume diets with some set meals varying in contents of fats and carbohydrates, they are efficient at compensating in their other meals to ensure they maintain average daily energy intakes (interestingly they did not compensate specifically for fats or carbohydrates, but generally ensured they obtained similar total calories each day regardless of nutrient types).

So, what about comparisons between people who are a normal weight and those who are overweight? Genetic factors can play a part, but to be brutally honest (as genetic factors cannot be changed) the most useful mentality is probably that this is one more challenge to overcome. It is not a reason to be overweight, but it might contribute and make losing weight harder than for other people.

Anyone who has a genetic predisposition to gaining weight is probably not reading this book to look for excuses, but to find some information that has a practical use. In other words, it is most appropriate to focus our attentions on what we can affect rather than what we cannot. If we were to gather a few dozen overweight individuals together and monitor their weight loss over time, some would lose weight quicker than others, and in some cases genetic factors would be involved in those differences. However, all could, and would, lose weight by adopting a healthy diet, increasing physical activity and eating less.

It has been found that overweight individuals are more likely to underestimate the energy content of a meal, and this may result in overweight people consuming larger meals[319,320]. Alternatively, it could be that lean individuals overestimate the energy content of meals as a protective mechanism to stay lean[320]. Curiously, if the same food carries a high-fat or low-fat label, this will affect how that food is perceived, with a 'high-fat' soup being perceived as more satisfying and creamy than the exact same soup with a 'low-fat' label. However, despite labels having an immediate effect on how a food is perceived, they have no effect on appetite half an hour after the meal is consumed[321].

Although many fad diets encourage individuals to increase intakes of some nutrients and reduce intakes of others, there are no differences in the overall effectiveness of these approaches over time, at least as far as fats and carbohydrates are concerned. The short-term effects of any energy-restricted diet include weight-loss and reduced cholesterol levels, but cholesterol will return to normal over time, and weight loss will only continue or be maintained by the careful management of an individual's energy balance. There are no significant differences between most diets, whether they are low-fat or low-carbohydrate, when considered in the longer term. However, high-protein diets have been shown to have some benefits over high-fat or high-carbohydrate ones ('high-protein' is about 35% of total energy intake).

* * * * * * *

One of the key adaptations to exercise is an increase in the amount of fat that is used for energy[322]. However, a further adaptation is an increase in fitness and energy-burning efficiency. That is, a given amount (duration and intensity) of exercise will use up more energy when someone starts to exercise, than that same exercise a few months later, once the individual has become adapted to it. So, for exercise to really contribute to weight-loss over time, it is necessary for the individual to continually increase the stimulus, by prolonging the duration or increasing the intensity of exercise, or both. Which kind of physical activity is really a matter for the individual, and the most important aspect of it is that it needs to be something the person is interested in. It does not matter if it is walking, jogging, cycling, a racket sport, a team sport or a computer-based fitness package. As long as it generates a sufficient physiological impact to require energy to be burned, then it will be useful. If exercise is comfortable, then it probably is not doing enough to use up much energy and promote weight loss, but for the sake of health nor should it be exasperating or painful[*].

Another matter of some relevance to this whole topic is the 'thermic effect of foods'. That is, how much a particular nutrient, food or meal increases metabolic rate. The digestive processes themselves have to use energy to work, and this energy loss can vary. Research has shown[323,324] that the thermic effect of a meal is not

---

[*] Anyone who is not used to exercising should be given a check by a doctor before beginning – just to ensure they are safe to start pushing themselves

significantly altered by the types of nutrients that comprise the meal, but is affected by the total energy content. This tends to be because meals are typically varied in their nutrient composition, making a meaningful analysis difficult. In difference to this, a recent review[323] reported that high-protein diets promoted the highest thermic effects and greatest levels of satiety. It was also reported that the thermic effect of a high-protein/low-fat meal is significantly greater than a high-carbohydrate/low-fat meal. For these reasons, a high-protein diet is usually recommended for people wishing to lose weight (35% protein, 35% carbohydrate, 30% fat).

Metabolic rate can be increased for several hours following a meal, even a fairly low-energy meal[324]. However, it has been found that obese individuals have a reduced thermic response[325]. This would mean that if someone lean and someone obese consumed identical meals, the obese person would use up less energy digesting it, and would therefore be more likely to have a positive energy balance if all other factors were equal. Hence, someone who is obese would have another challenge to weight-loss, greater than that of someone who is only slightly overweight.

So, calorie-counting is fairly meaningless, and it is the individual who best understands their dietary and lifestyle habits, and so is best placed to know what can be changed, which meals can be reduced, and how some sort of physical activity can best be introduced and/or increased. All the recommendations within this book are focussed on promoting good health and a lean body composition, because it is difficult to obtain too much energy from natural foods. The sorts of foods that contribute easily to a positive energy balance, and therefore weight-gain, are the high-energy, highly processed foods.

Even foods such as cereal grains and rice, because they are relatively high in energy and low in real nutrient content, are more likely to promote a positive energy balance than fruits and vegetables. Also, a diet rich in fruits, vegetables, meats and fish will contain all the nutrients a person needs in abundance, making it less likely they will suffer from food cravings that prevent weight-loss and lead to over-eating. So, a natural diet, which is naturally high in protein, fruits and vegetables, with plenty of physical exercise, is all that is really required to sustain a lean weight or promote weight loss. The science that supports this could be phenomenally complicated and involved, and many people would no doubt appreciate that, but it is admirably simple too, and has been summed-up sufficiently in this paragraph on the matter.

The real challenge is not the physiology of weight loss, which at best simply supports a high-protein intake (35% of total energy intake), plenty of fruits and vegetables, and increased physical activity. The challenge for most is the behavioural change required to consistently reduce meal size and increase physical activity over time. Everything is about the psychological needs of the individual, because the physiological needs are far simpler. Perhaps people attempt to over-complicate the physiological basis of weight-loss in order to compensate for the far more important, necessary and challenging aspects of the often over-looked psychological side.

Really, the primary focus should not be on targeting a specific amount of weight to lose, or a dress size to fit into. These are secondary aims and this is because they are actually quite negative. They are an end-result and until reached the goal has not been met, and each day of work and commitment passes perhaps for several weeks and even months without obtaining it. The foundation of effective, efficient and long-term, sustained weight-loss is commitment to a healthy diet and lifestyle, in which the body has all the nutrients required and does not suffer cravings for particular foods.

A healthy diet should be the primary focus, not only because it is the most important aspect of long-term weight-loss, but also because it does not require weeks or months of work – a healthier diet can be achieved within days, and satisfactorily improved upon over relatively short periods of time, hopefully with noticeable benefits in mood and general health. The only challenge is how to integrate and substitute in the healthier foods, so as to replace more common and less useful ones. This is a matter of taste and experimentation with recipes, and beyond that there is no further cause of delay. By aiming for health first the goal is quickly achieved, weight-loss becomes easier as a result, and life ought to feel better for the process.

* * * * * * *

Health is from the inside out, and does not and cannot work the other way around. Our modern focus on aesthetics and self-image has become somewhat misguided, not because there is anything wrong with wanting to be attractive and promote the self-image we want, but because we have been duped into thinking these require us to buy products and we cannot appear as we wish without them. Healthy-looking skin and hair requires a healthy body, with all the nutrients and care taken to promote total health. Cosmetics cover up, hide, fill-out and generally tamper with our appearance, rather than really nourishing our skin and nails in a healthy and supportive way. Not many people make money from healthy eating.

Assuming that being thin promotes a self-image of health is not true, and being thin certainly does not mean appearing attractive if the person is clearly unhealthy. Worst of all, that people focus on becoming a particular weight at the expense of their health is disastrous, although understandable due to modern media attentions and pressure. It leads to the implication that what people think of us is more important than our own health and well-being. It is intolerably superficial. If we forget about weight-loss supplements, about strategies and about media pressure, we can then focus on our real priority – ourselves.

Weight loss comes easiest with a diet that is inherently healthy, which by necessity does not generate cravings. There is no mileage in trying to trick the body into weight loss, in trying every single diet that ever comes along or paying for anything related to weight loss. A fully healthy self-image requires a fully selfish approach, in which we put our inner selves before the perception of ourselves by others. Rather than lose a good deal of weight in a couple of weeks, from which we would probably feel tired, lethargic and fatigued, we should aim to adopt a healthier diet and lifestyle, in which excess weight can be kept off for good. It might sound like rhetoric, but we have lost sight of the absolute basics because we imagine it is more complicated than it really is.

It is not complicated at all. It is incredibly simple: adopt a healthy diet. This will help most people lose some weight with no greater effort required. Promote further weight loss by increasing levels of physical activity. If the improved diet and increased physical activity have not already started a reasonable weight loss, then cut out any 'compromise' foods, such as cereal grain foods, including pasta, pastries and breads, as well as dairy and snack foods. Replace these entirely with fresh fruits and vegetables, and ensure a high-protein intake from fresh fish and meats. If, with diet optimal and the lifestyle active, more weight needs to be lost, then either reduce meal sizes or increase the intensity and/or duration of physical activity.

More energy has to be expended each day than is taken in. It is very simple, and it cannot be tricked. Nor can it fail – there is no possibility in human physiology that this simple approach can be anything but a success. It might be hard work, and it might take some time, but it will be worth it – a healthy body and healthy appearance are more worthwhile in the long-run than a two-week fix that causes more problems than it solves. The real focus needs to be on commitment to health first and foremost, with weight loss occurring far more easily as a result.

Final Thoughts

"If you have health, you probably will be happy, and if you have health and happiness, you have all the wealth you need, even if it is not all you want."

- Elbert Hubbard

It is time to abandon faith. It is time to abandon the grave misconception that people who invent diets do so out of any kind of altruistic drive. The diet industry, with all its books, articles, courses, special foods and magic pills, is a billion-dollar commercial enterprise, where the customer is the source of revenue, and the inventor the fat cat. The customers can be counted in their hundreds of millions, and all that fat cat needs is to sustain enough interest – enough short-term weight-loss in each of their customers – and the fat cat becomes fatter as the customer becomes pallid and depressed. It is time to realise that the one person who really cares most of all about you – about all of you – is you.

Perhaps you are fortunate enough to have close friends and family who you might include as an extension of who you are, but please do not imagine the CEO of your local supermarket or health food chain, or the government or even its health service, really cares about you as an individual. If anyone stands to make money out of you, then it is best to treat his or her advice with extreme, sceptical caution.

The human body is a biological organism that has been recognised in the fossil record for over two million years. The biological and environmental sciences have been employed effectively to describe with some accuracy how our bodies have evolved and adapted over its two-million-plus years of history. The human body is as simple or as complex as you wish to make it, depending upon the level of understanding you wish to have. Ultimately, however, everything comes down to simple processes.

The human body cannot be tricked by schemes, whether based upon sketchy science, pseudo-science, or just plain fashion. The body has no care for fashion, and is not interested in pseudo-science – the art of taking a piece of information and perverting it into often unrelated and abstract conjectures. But conjecture is all it turns out to be. It is not a theory, in the scientific sense of the word, and not even an hypothesis. It is mostly unfounded conjecture with the express intention of giving people a short-term return for the sake of commercial success, and often not for the reasons cited. By the time people have grown to find the diet unworkable, its creator has already made his or her fortune.

In fact, almost everything in this book has been superfluous, in that if you were to commit to a healthier diet and lifestyle you would not need this book. Most people would know to increase their consumption of fruits and vegetables, would probably have fish more often and limit their intake of red meat, preferring poultry and fish instead most days. We would also naturally increase our physical activity levels, and this is not a matter of joining a gym, but simply finding ways to be more active in everyday life: walking up and down escalators, taking stairs more than the lift, walking a bit further on a daily basis, and generally getting up and about more than usual. It all helps, and it is an important start – far more than signing money away on the hope a gym will do it for you. Go to the gym when you feel a need and desire to use those particular facilities to meet your goals, not because you think the gym is a solution in and of itself.

Mostly, this book has been about supporting what you

already know, and hopefully giving some additional information to guide decision-making. A few fruits and vegetables are better than none, but really we need to replace our cereal grain and dairy foods with them, recreating a more natural diet and promoting health and vitality for all the reasons cited here.

Some things were not covered and can be left to future editions when more information is available, but everything important should be found here. Cooking methods were not included much, although mostly because the initial focus should be on incorporating the right foods, with cooking methods being the fine-tuning that can come after. For the record, all foods should typically be cooked for the shortest period of time and at the lowest heat. Steaming is healthier than boiling, and frying meats and oils should be limited as much as possible. Meats and oils, including those in fish, should be heated minimally.

The microwave has received very bad press, but is probably the healthiest way to prepare foods. At the highest setting a microwave will break down nutrients too much, but on a medium setting a microwave will effectively heat the whole food throughout in a shorter time than any other type of cooking. With most cooking methods foods are heated from the outside to in, and by the time the food has been heated to its centre the outside has been overcooked and the nutrients damaged. This is avoided with a microwave, but only on a medium setting or below, which prevents the extent of damage to foods seen with the higher settings.

Oils in general should not be used to cook foods with, although this is obviously not necessary anyway with steaming or microwaving. Once heated, some oils become potentially harmful and even carcinogenic, and although olive and coconut oils are the most stable the effect still occurs, and olive oil should best be kept as a dressing. In any case, many vegetable oils contain high amounts of omega-6 fats, which should be included in the diet in levels roughly equivalent to those of the omega-3s.

Just because a particular food, or food processed or prepared in a particular way, increases the risk of some ill-effect, such as heart disease or cancer, this does not imply the effect occurs in everyone, or even in most people. Cancer and heart disease are the most common causes of premature death in the modern population, but not everyone will suffer from these. For a particular cancer or heart condition, only a small percentage of the population will suffer, and this book refers to the sorts of things that increase risk. The conditions cannot be prevented outright, but the risk of suffering from them can be reduced significantly in those wishing to be healthy. However, cancers happen naturally, and the focus is really to be less likely to suffer and more likely to recover if affected.

That some like to cite the person they knew who was always healthy yet died prematurely, or who did everything wrong but lived to a grand old age is not helpful. In research we might state that "data is not the plural of anecdote" because our personal experiences bias us to what has happened to a few hundred people at best. Population-based studies relate causes and effects amongst tens of thousands, or even hundreds of thousands of people, and then give a far fuller account of what affects health. Science is not overturned because one person knows of one person who was an exception, because the evidence clearly shows that exceptions, by definition, cannot represent the whole population. Science and medicine would be hopeless if this were otherwise. People who are interested in their health are more likely to live longer and enjoy better health, compared with people who are not – this is self-evident and platitudinous. There will be exceptions to this, but that does not mean we should be frivolous. Some people win the lottery and others get struck by lightning – exceptional things happen to people, but staking our health on the exceptions we know is unlikely to pay off.

Perhaps most importantly, by adopting a healthy diet – in which the body is better protected against harm – it is possible to have a few less healthy foods and not suffer ill-consequences. After all, it is repeated exposure that increases risk, and from a psychological perspective there is probably greater satisfaction in having them rarely rather than every day, and almost certainly better than avoiding them entirely. A healthy body cannot exist without a healthy mind – this can be associated with the effects of stress on the immune function and health of the cardiovascular system, metabolism and so on. The balance should be in favour of a healthy diet, with other foods included initially out of convenience during the transfer, but remaining rarely for the sake of any psychological needs.

"Live in rooms full of light
Avoid heavy food
Be moderate in the drinking of wine
Take massage, baths, exercise, and gymnastics
Fight insomnia with gentle rocking or the sound of running water
Change surroundings and take long journeys
Strictly avoid frightening ideas
Indulge in cheerful conversation and amusements
Listen to music."

- Aulus Cornelius Celsus
1st Century CE

Appendix

References

1. Cordain, L., Eaton, S. B., Sebastian, A., Mann, N., Lindeberg, S., Watkins, B. A., O'Keefe, J. H., Brand-Miller, J., "Origins and evolution of the Western diet: health implications for the 21st century", American Journal of Clinical Nutrition, 2005, 81, 341-354

2. Dietrich, C. G., Geier, A., Wasmuth, H. E., de Waart, D. R., Oude Elferink, R. P. J., Matern, S., Gartung, C., "Influence of biliary cirrhosis on the detoxification and elimination of a food derived carcinogen", Gut, 2004, 53, 1850-1855

3. Eastwood, M.A., Brydon, W.G., Anderson, D.M.W., "The effect of the polysaccharide composition and structure of dietary fibers on cecal fermentation and fecal excretion", The American Journal of Clinical Nutrition, 1986, 44, 51-55

4. Robertson, J., Brydon, W.G., Tadesse, K., Wenham, P., Walls, A., Eastwood, M.A., "The effect of raw carrot on serum lipids and colon function", American Journal of Clinical Nutrition, 1979, 32, 1889-1892

5. Lewis, M.J., Whorwell, P.J., "Bran: may irritate irritable bowel", Nutrition, 1998, 14(5), 470-471

6. Anderson, J.W., Gilinsky, N.H., Deakins, D.A., Smith, S.F., O'Neal, D.S., Dillon, D.W., Oeltgen, P.R., "Lipid responses of hypercholesterolemic men to oat-bran and wheat-bran intake", American Journal of Clinical Nutrition, 1991, 54, 678-683

7. Francis, C.Y., Whorwell, P.J., "Bran and irritable bowel syndrome: time for reappraisal", Lancet, 1994, 344(8914), 39-40

8. Reddy, K. S., Katan, M. B., "Diet, nutrition and the prevention of hypertension and cardiovascular diseases", Public Health Nutrition, 2004, 7 (1A), 167-186

9. Baer, D.J., Rumpler, W.V., Miles, C.W., Fahey, Jr., G.C., "Dietary fiber decreases the metabolizable energy content and nutrient digestibility of mixed diets fed to humans", Journal of Nutrition, 1997, 127, 579-586

10. Palafox-Carlos, H., Ayala-Zavala, J.F., Gonzalez-Aguilar, G.A., "The role of dietary fiber in the bioaccessibility and bioavailability of fruit and vegetable antioxidants", Journal of Food Science, 2011, 76(11), R6-R15

11. van het Hof, K.H., Brouwer, I.A., West, C.E., Haddeman, E., Steegers-Theunissen, R.P.M., van Dusseldorp, M., Weststrate, J.A., Eskes, T.K.A.B., Hautvast, J.G.A.J., "Bioavailability of lutein from vegetables is 5 times higher than that of beta-carotene", American Journal of Clinical Nutrition, 1999, 70, 261-268

12. Navarro Silvera, S.A., Mayne, S.T., Risch, H.A., Gammon, M.D., Vaughan, T., Chow, W.H., Dubin, J.A., Dubrow, R., Schoenberg, J., Stanford, J.L., West, A.B., Rotterdam, H., Blot, W.J., "Principle component analysis of dietary and lifestyle patterns in relation to risk of subtypes of oesophageal and gastric cancer", Annals of Epidemiology, 2011, March 23 (Epub)

13. Higdon, J.V., Delage, B., Williams, D.E., Dashwood, R.H., "Cruciferous vegetables and human cancer risk: Epidemiologic evidence and mechanistic basis", Pharmacological Research, 2007, 55(3), 224-236

14. Watzl, B., Bub, A., Briviba, K., Rechkemmer, G., "Supplementation of a low-carotenoid diet with tomato or carrot juice modulates immune functions in healthy

men", Annals of Nutrition and Metabolism, 2003, 47(6), 255-261

15. Yamazaki, M., Nishimura, T., "Induction of neutrophil accumulation by vegetable juice", Bioscience, Biotechnology and Biochemistry, 1992, 56(1), 150-151

16. Yamazaki, M., Ueda, H., Fukuda, K., Okamoto, M., Yui, S., "Priming effects of vegetable juice on endogenous production of tumor necrosis factor", Bioscience, Biotechnology and Biochemistry, 1992, 56(1), 149

17. Granado, F., Olmedilla, B., Herrero, C., Perez-Sacristan, B., Blanco, I., Blazquez, S., "Bioavailability of carotenoids and tocopherols from broccoli: in vivo and in vitro assessment", Experimental Biology and Medicine, 2006, 231, 1733-1738

18. Lotito, S.B., Frei, B., "Consumption of flavonoid-rich foods and increased plasma antioxidant capacity in humans: cause, consequence, or epiphenomenon?", Free Radical Biology and Medicine, 2006, 41(12), 1727-1746

19. Dehghan, M., Akhtar-Danesh, N., McMillan, C.R., Thabane, L., "Is plasma vitamin C an appropriate biomarker of vitamin C intake? A systematic review and meta-analysis", Nutrition Journal, 2007, 6, 41, Epub

20. Rasmussen, S.E., Breinholt, V.M., "Non-nutritive bioactive food constituents of plants: bioavailability of flavonoids", International Journal of Vitamin and Nutrient Research, 2003, 73(2), 101-111

21. van het Hof, K.H., West, C.E., Weststrate, J.A., Hautvast, J.G.A.J., "Dietary factors that affect the bioavailability of carotenoids", Journal of Nutrition, 2000, 130, 503-506

22. Edwards, A.J., You, C.-S., Swanson, J.E., Parker, R.S., "A novel extrinsic reference method for assessing the vitamin A value of plant foods", American Journal of Clinical Nutrition, 2001, 74, 348-355

23. Kiefer, I., Prock, P., Lawrence, C., Wise, J., Bieger, W., Bayer, P., Rathmanner, T., Kunze, M., Rieder, A., "Supplementation with mixed fruit and vegetable juice concentrates increased serum antioxidants and folate in healthy adults", Journal of the American College of Nutrition, 2004, 23(3), 205-211

24. Tyssandier, V., Reboul, E., Dumas, J.-F., Bouteloup-Demange, C., Armand, M., Marcand, J., Sallas, M., Borel, P., "Processing of vegetable-borne carotenoids in the human stomach and duodenum", American Journal of Physiology Gastrointestinal Liver Physiology, 2003, 284, G913-G923

25. Jonsson, L., "Thermal degradation of carotenes and influence on their physiological functions", Advances in Experimental Medicine and Biology, 1991, 289, 75-82

26. Gregory, J.F., "Ascorbic acid bioavailability in foods and supplements", Nutrition Reviews, 1993, 51(10), 301-303

27. Mangels, A.R., Block, G., Frey, C.M., Patterson, B.H., Taylor, P.R., Norkus, E.P., Levander, O.A., "The bioavailability to humans of ascorbic acid from oranges, orange juice and cooked broccoli is similar to that of synthetic ascorbic acid", Journal of Nutrition, 1993, 123, 1054-1061

28. Ryan, L., O'Connell, O., O'Sullivan, L., Aherne, S.A., O'Brien, N.M., "Micellarisation of carotenoids from raw and cooked vegetables", Plant Foods for Human Nutrition, 2008, 63(3), 127-133

29. O'Connell, O., Ryan, L., O'Sullivan, L., Aherne-Bruce, S.A., O'Brien, N.M., "Carotenoid micellarization varies greatly between individual and mixed vegetables with or without the addition of fat or fiber", International Journal for Vitamin and Nutrient Research, 2008, 78(4-5), 238-246

References

30. Tydeman, E.A., Parker, M.L., Faulks, R.M., Cross, K.L., Fillery-Travis, A., Gidley, M.J., Rich, G.T., Waldron, K.W., "Effect of carrot (Daucus carota) microstructure on carotene bioaccessibility in the upper gastrointestinal tract. 2. In vivo digestions", Journal of Agriculture and Food Chemistry, 2010, 58(17), 9855-9860

31. McEligot, A.J., Rock,C.L., Shanks, T.G., Flatt, S.W., Newman, V., Faerber, S., Pierce, J.P., "Comparison of serum carotenoid responses between women consuming vegetable juice and women consuming raw or cooked vegetables", Cancer Epidemiology, Biomarkers and Prevention, 1999, 8, 227-231

32. van het Hof, K.H., Tijburg, L.B., Pietrzik, K., Weststrate, J.A., "Influence of feeding different vegetables on plasma levels of carotenoids, folate and vitamin C. Effect of disruption of the vegetable matrix", British Journal of Nutrition, 1999, 82(3), 203-212

33. de Pee, S., West, C.E., Permaesih, D., Martuti, S Muhilal, Hautvast, J.G.A.J., "Orange fruit is more effective than are dark-green, leafy vegetables in increasing serum concentrations of retinol and beta-carotene in school children in Indonesia", American Journal of Clinical Nutrition, 1998, 68, 1058-1067

34. Hurrell, R.F., "Influence of vegetable protein sources on trace element and mineral bioavailability", Journal of Nutrition, 2003, 133, 2973S-2977S

35. Kopsell, D.A., Kopsell, D.E., "Accumulation and bioavailability of dietary carotenoids in vegetable crops", Trends in Plant Science, 2006, 11(10), 499-507

36. Livny, O., Reifen, R., Levy, I., Madar, Z., Faulks, R., Southon, S., Schwartz, B., "Beta-carotene bioavailability from differently processed carrot meals in human ileostomy volunteers", European Journal of Nutrition, 2003, 42(6), 338-345

37. Vermeulen, M., Klopping-Ketelaars, I.W., van den Berg, R., Vaes, W.H., "Bioavailability and kinetics of sulforaphane in humans after consumption of cooked versus raw broccoli", Journal of Agriculture and Food Chemistry, 2008, 56(22), 10505-10509

38. Griep, L.O., Verschuren, W.M., Kromhout, D., Ocke, M.C., Geleijnse, J.M., "Raw and processed fruit and vegetable consumption and 10-year stroke incidence in a population-based cohort study in the Netherlands", European Journal of Clinical Nutrition, 2011, March 23, Epub – doi:10.1038/ejcn.2011.36

39. Papetti, A., Daglia, M., Gazzani, G., "Anti- and pro-oxidant activity of water soluble compounds in Cichorium intybus var. silvestre (Treviso red chicory)", Journal of Pharmaceutical and Biomedicine Analysis, 2002, 30(4), 939-945

40. Tsai, H.C., Lee, S.S., Huang, C.K., Yen, C.M., Chen, E.R., Liu, Y.C., "Outbreak of eosinophilic meningitis assosciated with drinking raw vegetable juice in southern Taiwan", American Journal of Tropical Medicine and Hygeine, 2004, 71(2), 222-226

41. Song, H.P., Kim, D.H., Jo, C., Lee, C.H., Kim, K.S., Byun, M.W., "Effect of gamma irradiation on the microbiological quality and antioxidant activity of fresh vegetable juice", Food Microbiology, 2006, 23(4), 372-378

42. Smith, T.K., Mithen, R., Johnson, I.T., "Effects of brassica vegetable juice on the induction of apoptosis and aberrant crypt foci in rat colonic mucosal crypts in vivo", Carcinogenesis, 2003, 24(3), 491-495

43. Gill, C.I., Hadar, S., Boyd, L.A., Bennett, R., Whiteford, J., Butler, M., Pearson, J.R., Bradbury, I., Rowland, I.R., "Watercress supplementation in diet reduces lymphocyte DNA damage and alters blood antioxidant status in healthy adults", American Journal of Clinical Nutrition, 2007, 85(2), 504-510

44. Tang, L., Zirpoli, G.R., Guru, K., Moysich, K.B., Zhang, Y., Ambrosone, C.B.,

McCann, S.E., "Intake of cruciferous vegetables modifies bladder cancer survival", Cancer Epidemiology Biomarkers and Prevention, 2010, 19(7), 1806-1811

45. Intawongsee, M., Dean, J.R., "Uptake of heavy metals by vegetable plants grown on contaminated soil and their bioavailability in the human gastrointestinal tract", Food Additives and Contamination, 2006, 23(1), 36-48

46. Shenoy, S.F., Kazaks, A.G., Holt, R.R., Chen, H.J., Winters, B.L., Khoo, C.S., Poston, W.S.C., Haddock, C.K., Reeves, R.S., Foreyt, J.P., Gershwin, M.E., Keen, C.L., "The use of a commercial vegetable use as a practical means to increase vegetable intake: a randomized controlled trial", Nutrition Journal, 2010, 9, 38, Epub

47. Fan, W.Y., Ogusu, K., Kouda, K., Nakamura, H., Satoh, T., Ochi, H., Takeuchi, H., "Reduced oxidative DNA damage by vegetable juice intake: A controlled trial", Journal of Physiological Anthropology and Applied Human Science, 2000, 19(6), 287-289

48. Hadley, C.W., Clinton, S.K., Schwartz, S.J., "The consumption of processed tomato products enhances plasma lycopene concentrations in association with a reduced lipoprotein sensitivity to oxidative damage", Journal of Nutrition, 2003, 133, 727-732

49. Kong, F., Singh, R.P., "Solid loss of carrots during simulated gastric digestion", Food Biophysics, 2011, 6, 84-93

50. Sarwar, G., Peace, R.W., "Comparisons between true digestibility of total nitrogen and limiting amino acids in vegetable proteins fed to rats", Journal of Nutrition, 1986, 116, 1172-1184

51. Noakes, M., Keogh, J.B., Foster, P.R., Clifton, P.M., "Effect of an energy-restricted, high-protein, low-fat diet relative to a conventional high-carbohydrate, low-fat diet on weight loss, body composition, nutritional status, and markers of cardiovascular health in obese women", American Journal of Clinical Nutrition, 2005, 81(6), 1298-1306

52. Clifton, P.M., Bastiaans, K., Keogh, J.B., "High protein diets decrease total and abdominal fat and improve CVD risk profile in overweight and obese men and women with elevated triacylclyerol", Nutrition, Metabolism and Cardiovascular Diseases, 2009, 19(8), 548-554

53. Iso, H., Stampfer, M.J., Manson, J.E., Rexrode, K., Hu, F., Hennekens, C.H., Colditz, G.A., Speizer, F.E., Willett, W.C., "Prospective study of fat and protein intake and risk of intraparenchymal hemorrhage in women", Circulation, 2001, 103(6), 856-863

54. Preis, S.R., Stampfer, M.J., Spiegelman, D., Willett, W.C., Rimm, E.B., "Lack of association between dietary protein intake and risk of stroke among middle-aged men", American Journal of Clinical Nutrition, 2010, 91(1), 39-45

55. Larsson, S.C., Virtamo, J., Wolk, A., "Red meat consumption and risk of stroke in Swedish women", Stroke, 2011, 42(2), 324-329

56. Babio, N., Sorli, M., Bulló, M., Basora, J., Ibarrola-Jurado, N., Fernández-Ballart, J., Martinez-González, M.A., Serra-Majem, L., González-Pérez, R., Salas-Salvadó, J., on behalf of the Nureta-PREDIMED investigators, "Association between red meat consumption and metabolic syndrome in a Mediterranean population at high cardiovascular risk: Cross-sectional and 1-year follow-up assessment", Nutrition, Metabolism, and Cardiovascular Diseases, 2010, September 26 (Epub)

57. Azadbakht, L., Esmaillzadeh, A., "Red meat intake is associated with metabolic syndrome and the plasma c-reactive protein concentration in women", The Journal of Nutrition, 2009, 139, 335-339

References

58. McAfee, A.J., McSorley, E.M., Cuskelly, G.J., Fearon, A.M., Moss, B.W., Beattie, J.A., Wallace, J.M., Bonham, M.P., Strain, J.J., "Red meat from animals offered a grass diet increases plasma and platelet n-3 PUFA in healthy consumers", British Journal of Nutrition, 2011, 105(1), 80-89

59. Villaverde, C., Baucells, M.D., Cortinas, L., Hervera, M., Barroeta, A.C., "Chemical composition and energy content of chickens in response to different levels of dietary polyunsaturated fatty acids", Archives of Animal Nutrition, 2005, 59(4), 281-292

60. Bevacqua, C.E., Rice, C.P., Torrents, A., Ramirez, M., "Steroid hormones in bio solids and poultry litter: A comparison of potential environmental inputs", The Science of the Total Environment, 2011, 409(11), 2120-2126

61. Divari, S., Cannizzo, F.T., Uslenghi, F., Pregel, P., Mulasso, C., Spada, F., De Maria, R., Biolatti, B., "Corticosteroid hormone receptors and prereceptors as new biomarkers of the illegal use of glucocorticoids in meat production", Journal of Agricultural and Food Chemistry, 2011, 59(5), 2120-2125

62. Scarth, J., Akre, C., van Ginkel, L., Le Bizec, B., De Brabander, H., Korth, W., Points, J., Teale, P., Kay, J., "Presence and metabolism of endogenous androgenic-anabolic steroid hormones in meat-producing animals: a review", Food Additives and Contaminants. Part A Chemistry, analysis, control, exposure and risk assessment, 2009, 26(5), 640-671

63. Castanon, J.I.R., "History of the use of antibiotic as growth promoters in European poultry feeds", Poultry Science, 2007, 86, 2466-2471

64. Vignaroli, C., Zandri, G., Aquilanti, L., Pasquaroli, S., Biavasco, F., "Multidrug-resistant enterococci in animal meat and faeces and co-transfer of resistance from an Enterococcus durans to a human Enterococcus faecium", Current Microbiology, 2011, 62(5), 1438-1447

65. Dhanarani, T.S., Shankar, C., Park, J., Dexilin, M., Rajesh Kumar, R., Thamaraiselvi, K., "Study on acquisition of bacterial antibiotic resistance determinants in poultry litter", Poultry Science, 2009, 88, 1381-1387

66. Huber, H., Ziegler, D., Pflüger, V., Vogel, G., Zweifel, C., Stephan, R., "Prevalence and characteristics of methicillin-resistant coagulase-negative staphylococci from livestock, chicken carcasses, bulk tank milk, minced meat, and contact persons", BMC Veterinary Research, 2011, 7(6) (Epub)

67. Gill, J.L., Bishop, S.C., McCorquodale, C., Williams, J.L., Wiener, P., "Association of selected SNP with carcass and taste panel assessed meat quality traits in a commercial population of Aberdeen Angus-sired beef cattle", Genetics Selection Evolution, 2009, 41(36) (Epub)

68. Wright, J.L., Neuhouser, M.L., Lin, D.W., Kwon, E.M., Feng, Z., Ostrander, E.A., Stanford, J.L., "AMACR polymorphisms, dietary intake of red meat and dairy and prostate cancer risk", Prostate, 2011, 71(5), 498-506

69. Cross, A.J., Freedman, N.D., Ren, J., Ward, M.H., Hollenbeck, A.R., Schatzkin, A., Sinha, R., Abnet, C.C., "Meat consumption and risk of esophageal and gastric cancer in a large prospective study", American Journal of Gastroenterology, 2011, 106(3), 432-442

70. Creton, S.K., Zhu, H., Gooderham, N.J., "The cooked meat carcinogen 2-amino-1-methyl-6-phenylimidazo[4,5-b]pyridine activates the extracellular signal-regulated kinase mitogen-activated protein kinase pathway", Cancer Research, 2007, 67(23), 11455-11462

71. Lauber, S.N., Gooderham, N.J., "The cooked meat-derived genotoxic carcinogen 2-amino-3-methylimidazo[4,5-b]pyridine has potent hormone-like activity: Mechanistic support for a role in breast cancer", Cancer Research, 2007, 67(19), 9597-9602

72. Alaejos, M.S., González, V., Afonso, A.M., "Exposure to heterocyclic aromatic amines from the consumption of cooked red meat and its effect on human cancer risk: a review", Food Additives and Contaminants. Part A Chemistry, analysis, control, exposure and risk assessment, 2008, 25(1), 2-24

73. Gorelik, S., Ligumsky, M., Kohen, R., Kanner, J., "The stomach as a "biomarker": when red meat meets red wine", Journal of Agricultural and Food Chemistry", 2008, 56, 5002-5007

74. Cho, E., Chen, W.Y., Hunter, D.J., Stampfer, M.J., Colditz, G.A., Hankinson, S.E., Willett, W.C., "Red meat intake and risk of breast cancer among premenopausal women", Archives of Internal Medicine, 2006, 166, 2253-2259

75. Linos, E., Willett, W.C., Cho, E., Colditz, G., Frazier, L.A., "Red meat consumption during adolescence among premenopausal women and risk of breast cancer", Cancer Epidemiology, Biomarkers and Prevention, 2008, 17(8), 2146-2151

76. Williams, C.D., Satia, J.A., Adair, L.S., Stevens, J., Galanko, J., Keku, T.O., Sandler, R.S., "Associations of red meat, fat, and protein intake with distal colorectal cancer risk", Nutrition and Cancer, 2010, 62(6), 701-709

77. Alexander, D.D., Weed, D.L., Cushing, C.A., Lowe, K.A., "Meta-analysis of prospective studies of red meat consumption and colorectal cancer", European Journal of Cancer Prevention, 2011, May 2 (Epub).

78. Cotterchio, M., Boucher, B.A., Manno, M., Gallinger, S., Okey, A.B., Harper, P.A., "Red meat intake, doneness, polymorphisms in genes that encode carcinogen-metabolizing enzymes, and colorectal cancer risk", Cancer Epidemiological Biomarkers and Prevention, 2008, 17(11), 3098-3107

79. Joshi, A.D., Corral, R., Siegmund, K.D., Haile, R.W., Le Marchand, L., Martínez, M.E., Ahnen, D.J.,

80. Toden, S., Bird, A.R., Topping, D.L., Conlon, M.A., "High red meat diets induce greater numbers of colonic DNA double-strand breaks than white meat in rats: attenuation by high-amylose maize starch", Carcinogenesis, 2007, 28(11), 2355-2362

81. Sinha, R., Cross, A.J., Graubard, B.I., Leitzmann, M.F., Schatzkin, A., "Meat intake and mortality: a prospective study of over half a million people", Archives of Internal Medicine, 2009, 169(6), 562-571

82. Joosen, A.M.C.P., Kuhnle, G.G.C., Aspinall, S.M., Barrow, T.M., Lecommandeur, E., Azqueta, A., Collins, A.R., Bingham, S.A., "Effect of processed and red meat on endogenous nitrosation and DNA damage", Carcinogenesis, 2009, 30(8), 1402-1407

83. Santarelli, R.L., Vendeuvre, J.L., Naud, N., Taché, S., Guéraud, F., Viau, M., Genot, C., Corpet, D.E., Pierre, F.H., "Meat processing and colon carcinogenesis: cooked, nitrite-treated, and oxidized high-heme cured meat promotes mucin-depleted foci in rats", Cancer Prevention Research (Phila), 2010, 3(7), 852-864

84. Kuhnle, G.G., Story, G.W., Reda, T., Mani, A.R., Moore, K.P., Lunn, J.C., Bingham, S.A., "Diet-induced endogenous formation of nitroso compounds in the GI tract", Free Radical Biology and Medicine, 2007, 43(7), 1040-1047

85. Hodgson, J.M., Ward, N.C., Burke, V., Beilin, L.J., Puddey, I.B., "Increased lean red meat intake does not elevate markers of oxidative stress and inflammation in humans", The Journal of Nutrition, 2007, 137, 363-367

References

86. Dyall, S.C., "Methodological issues and inconsistencies in the field of omega-3 fatty acids research", Prostaglandins, Leukotrienes, and Essential Fatty Acids, 2011, 85(5), 281-285

87. Grootveld, M., Atherton, M.D., Sheerin, A.N., Hawkes, J., Blake, D.R., Richens, T.E., Silwood, C.J., Lynch, E., Claxson, A.W., "In vivo absorption, metabolism, and urinary excretion of alpha, beta-unsaturated aldehydes in experimental animals. Relevance to the development of cardiovascular diseases by the dietary ingestion of thermally stressed polyunsaturated-rich culinary oils", Journal of Clinical Investigation, 1998, 101(6), 1210-1218

88. Raff, M., Tholstrup, T., Basu, S., Nonboe, P., Sorensen, M.T., Straarup, E.M., "A diet rich in conjugated linoleic acid and butter increases lipid per oxidation but does not affect atherosclerotic, inflammatory, or diabetic risk markers in healthy young men", The Journal of Nutrition, 2008, 138, 509-514

89. Sotiroudis, T.G., Kyrtopoulos, S.A., "Anticarcinogenic compounds of olive oil and related biomarkers", European Journal of Nutrition, 2008, 47(Supplement 2), 69-72

90. Dyall, S.C., Michael-Titus, A.T., "Neurological benefits of omega-3 fatty acids", Neuromolecular Medicine, 2008, 10(4), 219-235

91. Weir, E., "Sushi, nemotodes and allergies", Canadian Medical Association Journal, 2005, 172(3), 329

92. Mol, S., "Levels of heavy metals in canned bonito, sardines, and mackerel produced in Turkey", Biological Trace Element Research, 2010, Dec 1 (Epub ahead of print)

93. Mol, S., "Determination of trace metals in canned anchovies and canned rainbow trouts", Food and Chemical and Toxicology, 2011, 49(2), 348-351

94. Ashraf, W., Seddigi, Z., Abulkibash, A., Khalid, M., "Levels of selected metals in canned fish consumed in Kingdom of Saudi Arabia", Environmental Monitoring and Assessment, 2006, 117(1-3), 271-279

95. Burger, J., Gochfeld, M., "Mercury in canned tuna: white versus light and temporal variation", Environmental Research, 2004, 96(3), 238-249

96. Xue, F., Holzman, C., Rahbar, M.H., Trosko, K., Fischer, L., "Maternal fish consumption, mercury levels, and risk of preterm delivery", Environmental Health Perspectives, 2007, 115(1), 42-47

97. Kipcić, D., Vukusić, J., "Polychlorinated biphenyls in fresh and canned fish from the Central Adriatic", Food Additives and Contaminants, 1991, 8(4), 501-504

98. Simoneau, C., Theobald, A., Hannaert, P., Roncari, P., Roncari, A., Rudolph, T., Anklam, E., "Monitoring of biphenyl-A-diglycidyl-ether (BADGE) in canned fish in oil", Food Additives and Contaminants, 1999, 16(5), 189-195

99. Simoneau, C., Theobald, A., Wiltschko, D., Anklam, E., "Estimation of intake of biphenyl-A-diglycidyl-ether (BADGE) from canned fish consumption in Europe and migration survey, 1999, 16(11), 457-463

100. Theobald, A., Simoneau, C., Hannaert, P., Roncari, P., Roncari, A., Rudolph, T., Anklam, E., "Occurrence of biphenyl-F-diglycidyl ether (BFDGE) in fish canned in oil", Food Additives and Contaminants, 2000, 17(10), 881-887

101. Fay, L.B., Leaf, C.D., Gremaud, E., Aeschlimann, J-M., Steen, C., Shuker, D.E.G., Turesky, R.J., "Urinary excretion of 3-methyl adenine after consumption of fish containing high levels of dim ethylamine", Carcinogenesis, 1997, 18(5), 1039-1044

102. Navas-Carretero, S., Perez-Granados, A.M., Schoppen, S., Vaquero, M.P., "An oily fish diet increases insulin sensitivity compared to a red meat diet in young iron-

deficient women", British Journal of Nutrition, 2009, 102(4), 546-553

103. Navas-Carretero, S., Perez-Granados, A.M., Schoppen, S., Sarria, B., Carbajal, A., Vaquero, M.P., "Iron status biomarkers in iron deficient women consuming oily fish versus red meat diet", Journal of Physiology and Biochemistry, 2009, 65(2), 165-174

104. Gao, Q., Niti, M., Feng, L., Yap, K.B., Ng, T.P., "Omega-3 polyunsaturated fatty acid supplements and cognitive decline: Singapore longitudinal aging studies", Journal of Nutrition, Health and Aging, 2011, 15(1), 32-35

105. Bousquet, M., Saint-Pierre, M., Julien, C., Salem Jr, N., Cicchetti, F., Calon, F., "Beneficial effects of dietary omega-3 polyunsaturated fatty acid on toxin-induced neuronal degeneration in an animal model of Parkinson's disease", The FASEB Journal, 2008, 22, 1213-1225

106. Gladyshev, M.I., Sushchik, N.N., Makhutova, O.N., Kalachova, G.S., "Content of essential polyunsaturated fatty acids in three canned fish species", International Journal of Food Sciences and Nutrition, 2009, 60(3), 224-230

107. Goldman, J.M., Murr, A.S., Buckalew, A.R., Ferrell, J.M., Cooper, R.L., "Moderating influence of the drinking water disinfection by-product dibromoacetic acid on a dithiocarbamate-induced suppression of the luteinizing hormone surge in female rats", Reproductive toxicology, 2007, 23(4), 541-549

108. Garofalo, R., "Cytokines in human milk", Journal of Pediatrics, 2010, 156(2 Supplement), S36-S40

109. Oddy, W.H., Rosales, F., "A systematic review of the importance of milk TGF-beta on immunological outcomes in the infant and young child", Pediatric Allergy and Immunology, 2010. 21, 47-59

110. Kunz, C., Rudolf, S., "Potential anti-inflammatory and anti-infectious effects of human milk oligosaccharides", Advances in Experimental Medicine and Biology, 2008, 606, 455-465

111. Hosea Blewett, H.J., Cicalo, M.C., Holland, C.D., Field, C.J., "The immunological compounds of human milk", Advances in Food and Nutrition Research, 2008, 54, 45-80

112. Lopez-Exposito, I., Recio, I., "Protective effect of milk peptides: antibacterial and antitumor properties", Advances in Experimental Medicine and Biology, 2008, 606, 271-293

113. Ogra, P.L., "Developmental aspects of the mucosal immune system: role of external environment, mucosal microflora and milk", Advances in Experimental Medicine and Biology, 2009, 639, 41-56

114. Manz, F., "Why is the phosphorous content of human milk exceptionally low?", Monatsschrift Kinderheilkunde, 1992, 140(9 Supplement 1), S35-S39

115. Powe, C.E., Knott, C.D., Conklin-Brittain, N., "Infant sex predicts breast milk energy content", American Journal of Human Biology, 2010, 22(1), 50-54

116. Anderson, G.H., Atkinson, S.A., Bryan, M.H., "Energy and macronutrient content of human milk during early lactation from mothers giving birth prematurely and at term", American Journal of Clinical Nutrition, 1981, 34, 258-265

117. Hosoi, S., Honma, K., Daimatsu, T., Kiyokawa, M., Aikawa, T., Watanabe, S., "Lower energy content of human milk than calculated using conversion factors", Pediatrics International, 2005, 47(1), 7-9

118. Hoppe, C., Andersen, G.S., Jacobsen, S., Molgaard, C., Friis, H., Sangild, P.T., Michaelsen, K.F., "The use of whey or skimmed milk powder in fortified blended foods for vulnerable groups", Journal of Nutrition, 2008, 138, 145S-161S

References

119. Heaney, R.P., "Calcium, dairy products and osteoporosis", Journal of the American College of Nutrition, 2000, 19(2), 83S-99S

120. Luopajärvi, K., Savilaht, E., Virtanen, S.M., Ilonen, J., Knip, M., Akerblom, H.K., Vaarala, O., "Enhanced levels of cow's milk antibodies in infancy in children who develop type 1 diabetes later in childhood", Pediatric Diabetes, 2009, 9(5), 434-441

121. Lanou, A.J., "Should dairy be recommended as part of a healthy vegetarian diet? Counterpoint", American Journal of Clinical Nutrition, 2009, 89(Supplement), 1638S-1642S

122. Lanou, A.J., Berkow, S.E., Barnard, N.D., "Calcium, dairy products, and bone health in children and young adults: A reevaluation of the evidence", Pediatrics, 2005, 115(3), 736-743

123. Merrilees, M.J., Smart, E.J., Gilchrist, N.L., Frampton, C., Turner, J.G., Hooke, E., March, R.L., Maguire, P., "Effects of dairy food supplements on bone mineral density in teenage girls", European Journal of Nutrition, 2000, 39(6), 256-262

124. Gibbons, M.J., Gilchrist, N.L., Frampton, C., Maguire, P., Reilly, P.H., March, R.L., Wall, C.R., "The effects of a high calcium dairy food on bone health in pre-pubertal children in New Zealand", Asia Pacific Journal of Clinical Nutrition, 2004, 13(4), 341-347

125. Basnet, S., Schneider, M., Gazit, A., Mander, G., Doctor, A., "Fresh goat's milk for infants: Myths and realities - a review", Pediatrics, 2010, 125(4), E973-E977

126. Carvalho, N.F., Kenney, R.D., Carrington, P.H., Hall, D.E., "Severe nutritional deficiencies in toddlers resulting from health food milk alternatives", Pediatrics, 2001, 107(4), 1-7

127. Ma, D., Jones, G., "Soft drink and milk consumption, physical activity, bone mass, and upper limb fractures in children: a population-based case-control study", Calcified Tissue International, 2004, 75(4), 286-291

128. Kalkwarf, H.J., Khoury, J.C., Lanphear, B.P., "Milk intake during childhood and adolescence, adult bone density, and osteoporotic fractures in US women", American Journal of Clinical Nutrition, 2003, 77, 257-265

129. Melnik, B.C., Schmitz, G., "Role of insulin, insulin-like growth factor-1, hyperglycaemic food and milk consumption in the pathogenesis of acne vulgaris", Experimental Dermatology, 2009, 18(10), 833-841

130. Qin, L.Q., He, K., Xu, J.Y., "Milk consumption and circulating insulin-like growth factor-I level: a systematic literature review", International Journal of Food Science and Nutrition, 2009, 60 (Supplement 7), 330-340

131. Newmark, H.L., Heaney, R.P., "Dairy products and prostate cancer risk", Nutrition and Cancer, 2010, 62(3), 297-299

132. Hjartaker, A., Thoresen, M., Engeset, D., Lund, E., "Dairy consumption and calcium intake and risk of breast cancer in a prospective cohort: The Norwegian Women and Cancer study", Cancer Causes Control, 2010, 21, 1875-1885

133. Huncharek, M., Muscat, J., Kupelnick, B., "Colorectal cancer risk and dietary intake of calcium, vitamin D, and dairy products: a meta-analysis of 26,335 cases from 60 observational studies", Nutrition and Cancer, 2009, 61(1), 47-69

134. Feskanich, D., Willett, W.C., Colditz, G.A., "Calcium, vitamin D, milk consumption, and hip fractures: a prospective study among postmenopausal women", American Journal of Clinical Nutrition, 2003, 77, 504-511

135. van Beresteijn, E.C.H., Brussaard, J.H., van Schaik, M., "Relationship between

the calcium-to-protein ratio in milk and the urinary calcium excretion in health adults - a controlled crossover study", American Journal of Clinical Nutrition, 1990, 52, 142-146

136. Lester, G., "Bone quality: Summary of NIH/ASBMR meeting", Journal of Musculoskeletal Neuronal Interactions, 2005, 5(4), 309

137. Gafni, R.I., Baron, J., "Childhood bone mass acquisition and peak bone mass may not be important determinants of bone mass in late adulthood", Pediatrics, 2007, 119 (Supplement 2), S131-S136

138. Bacciottini, L., Tanini, A., Falchetti, A., Masi, L., Franceschelli, F., Pampaloni, b., Giorgi, G., Brandi, M.L., "Calcium bioavailability from a calcium-rich mineral water, with some observations on method", Journal of Clinical Gastroenterology, 2004, 38(9), 761-766

139. Wynn, E., Raetz, E., Burckhardt, P., "The composition of mineral waters sourced from Europe and North America in respect to bone health: composition of mineral water optimal for bone", British Journal of Nutrition, 2009, 101(8), 1195-1199

140. Wynn, E., Krieg, M.A., Aeschlimann, J.M., Burckhardt, P., "Alkaline mineral water lowers bone resorption even in calcium sufficiency: alkaline mineral water and bone metabolism", Bone, 2009, 44(1), 120-124

141. New, S.A., "Nutrition Society Medal lecture. The role of the skeleton in acid-base homestasis", Proceedings of the Nutrition Society, 2002, 61(2), 151-164

142. Arnett, T.R., "Extracellular pH regulates bone cell function", The Journal of Nutrition, 2008, 138, 415S-418S

143. Frassetto, L.A., Morris, R.C.Jr., Sebastian, A., "Dietary sodium chloride intake independently predicts the degree of hyperchloremic metabolic acidosis in healthy humans consuming a net acid-producing diet", American Journal of Physiology. Renal Physiology, 2007, 293, F521-F525

144. Lemann, J. Jr., Adams, N.D., Wilz, D.R., Brenes, L.G., "Acid and mineral balances and bone in familial proximal renal tubular acidosis", Kidney International, 2000, 58(3), 1267-1277

145. Moe, O.W., Huang, C.L., "Hypercalciuria from acid load: renal mechanisms", Journal of Nephrology, 2006, 19 (Supplement 9), S53-S61

146. Zhang, L., Curhan, G.C., Forman, J.P., "Diet-dependent net acid load and risk of incident hypertension in US women", Hypertension, 2009, 54(4), 751-755

147. Cogan, M.G., Carneiro, A.V., Tatsuno, J., Colman, J., Krapf, R., Morris, R.C.Jr., Sebastian, A., "Normal diet NaCl variation can affect the renal set-point for plasma pH-(HCO_3^-) maintenance", Journal of the American Society of Nephrology, 1990, 1, 193-199

148. Lemann, J.Jr., Bushinsky, D.A., Hamm, L.L., "Bone buffering of acid and base in humans", American Journal of Physiology. Renal Physiology, 2003, 285, F811-F832

149. Neuman, M.W., Imai, K., Kawase, T., Saito, S., "The calcium-buffering phase of bone mineral: some clues to its form and formation", Journal of Bone and Mineral Research, 1987, 2(3), 171-181

150. Cao, J.J., Nielsen, F.H., "Acid diet (high-meat protein) effects on calcium metabolism and bone health", Current Opinions in Clinical Nutrition and Metabolic Care, 2010, 13(6), 698-702

151. Bushinsky, D.A., Smith, S.B., Gavrilov, K.L., Gavrilov, L.F., Li, J., Levi-Setti, R., "Acute acidosis-induced alternation in bone bicarbonate and phosphate", Americal Journal of Physiology. Renal Physiology, 2002, 283, F1091-F1097

References

152. Arnett, T., "Regulation of bone cell formation by acid-base balance", Proceedings of the Nutrition Society, 2003, 62(2), 511-520

153. Krieger, N.S., Frick, K.K., Bushinsky, D.A., "Mechanism of acid-induced bone resorption", Current Opinion in Nephrology and Hypertension, 2004, 13(4), 423-436

154. Bushinsky, D.A., "Acid-base imbalance and the skeleton", European Journal of Nutrition, 2001, 40(5), 238-244

155. Bushinsky, D.A., Smith, S.B., Gavrilov, K.L., Gavrilov, L.F., Li, J., Levi-Setti, R., "Chronic acidosis-induced alternation in bone bicarbonate and phosphate", Americal Journal of Physiology. Renal Physiology, 2003, 285, F532-F539

156. Bushinsky, D.A., "Contribution of organic material to the ion composition of bone", Journal of Bone and Mineral Research, 2000, 15(10), 2026-2032

157. Burton, R.F., "The roles of intracellular buffers and bone mineral in the regulation of acid-base balance in mammals", Comparative Biochemistry and Physiology. Comparative Physiology. 1992, 102(3), 425-432

158. Bushinsky, D.A., Chabala, J.M., Gavrilov, K.L., Levi-Setti, R., "Effects of in vivo metabolic acidosis on midcortical bone ion composition", American Journal of Physiology. Renal Physiology, 1999, 277, F813-J819

159. Freudiger, H., Bonjour, J.P., "Bisphosphonates and extrarenal acid buffering capacity", Calcified Tissue International, 1989, 44(1), 3-10

160. Wagner, E.A., Falciglia, G.A., Amlal, H., Levin, L., Soleimani, M., "Short-term exposure to a high-protein diet differentially affects glomerular filtration rate but not acid-base balance in older compared to younger adults", Journal of the American Dietetic Association, 2007, 107(8), 1404-1408

161. Domrongkitchaiporn, S., Pongskul, C., Sirikulchayanonta, V., Stitchantrakul, W., Leeprasert, V., Ongphiphadhanakul, B., Radinahamed, P., Rajatanavin, R., "Bone histology and bone mineral density after correction of acidosis in distal renal tubular acidosis", Kidney International, 2002, 62(6), 2160-2166

162. Siener, R., Jahnen, A., Hesse, A., "Influence of a mineral water rich in calcium, magnesium and bicarbonate on urine composition and the risk of calcium oxalate crystallization", European Journal of Clinical Nutrition, 2004, 58(2), 279-276

163. Verhas, M., de La Guéronnière, V., Grognet, J-M., Paternot, J., Hermanne, A., Van den Winkel, P., Gheldof, R., Martin, P., Fantino, M., Rayssiguier, Y., "Magnesium bioavailability from mineral water. A study in adult men". European Journal of Clinical Nutrition, 2002, 56, 442-447

164. Kiss, S., A., Forster, T., Dongo, A., "Absorption and effect of the magnesium content of a mineral water in the human body", Journal of the American College of Nutrition, 2004, 23(6), 758S-762S

165. Rylander, R., Arnaud, M.J., "Mineral water intake reduces blood pressure among subjects with low urinary magnesium and calcium levels", BMC Public Health, 2004, 4(56), 1-5

166. Guillemant, J., Le, H.-T., Accarie, C., du Montcel, S. T., Delabroise, A.-M., Arnaud, M. J., Guillemant, S., "Mineral water as a source of dietary calcium: acute effects on parathyroid function and bone resorption in young men", American Journal of Clinical Nutrition, 2000, 71, 999-1002

167. Burckhardt, P., "The effect of the alkali load of mineral water on bone metabolism: Interventional studies", The Journal of Nutrition, 2008, 138, 435S-437S

168. Loy, A., Beisker, W., Meier, H., "Diversity of bacteria growing in natural mineral water after bottling", Applied and Environmental Microbiology, 2005, 71(7),

3624-3632

169. Pinto, B., Reali, D., "Screening of estrogen-like activity of mineral water stored in PET bottles", International Journal of Hygeine and Environmental Health", 2009, 212(2), 228-232

170. Montuori, P., Jover, E., Morgantini, M., Bayona, J.M., Triassi, M., "Assessing human exposure to phthalic acid and phthalate esters from mineral water stored in polyethylene terephthalate and glass bottles", Food Additives & Contaminants Part A Chemistry, Analysis, Control, Exposure & Risk Assessment, 2008, 25(4), 511-518

171. Wagner, M., Oehlmann, J., "Endocrine disrupters in bottled mineral water: total estrogenic burden and migration from plastic bottles", Environmental Science and Pollution Research International, 2009., 16(3), 278-286

172. Darowska, A., Borcz, A., Nawrocki, J., "Aldehyde contamination of mineral water stored in PET bottles", Food Additives & Contaminants, 2003, 20(12), 1170-1177

173. Biscardi, D., Monarca, S., De Fusco, R., Senatore, F., Poli, P., Buschini, A., Rossi, C., Zani, C., "Evaluation of the migration of mutragens/carcinogens from PET bottles into mineral water by Tradescantia/micronuclei test, Comet assay on leukocytes and GC/MS", The Science of the Total Environment, 2003, 302 (1-3), 101-108

174. Willershausen, B., Kroes, H., Brandenbusch, M., "Evaluation of the contents of mineral water, spring water, table water and spa water", European Journal of Medical Research, 2000, 5(6), 251-262

175. York, R.G., Funk, K.A., Girard, M.F., Mattie, D., Strawson, J.E., "Oral (drinking water) developmental toxicity study of ammonium perchlorate in Sprague-Dawley rats", International Journal of Toxicology, 2003, 22(6), 453-464

176. Siglin, J.C., Mattie, D.R., Dodd, D.E., Hildebrandt, P.K., Baker, W.H., "A 90-day drinking water toxicity study in rats of the environmental contaminant ammonium perchlorate", Toxicological Science, 2000, 57, 61-74

177. Brechner, R.J., Parkhurst, G.D., Humble, W.O., Brown, M.B., Herman, W.H., "Ammonium perchlorate contamination of Colorado River drinking water is associated with abnormal thyroid function in newborns in Arizona", Journal of Occupational and Environmental Medicine, 2000, 42(8), 777-782

178. Steinmaus, C., Miller, M.D., Smith, A.H., "Perchlorate in drinking water during pregnancy and neonatal thyroid hormone levels in California", Journal of Occupational and Environmental Medicine, 2010, 52(1), 1217-1224

179. Blount, B.C., Alwis, K.U., Jain, R.B., Solomon, B.L., Morrow, J.C., Jackson, W.A., "Perchlorate, nitrate, and iodide intake through tap water", Environmental Science and Technology, 2010, 44(24), 9564-9570

180. Buffler, P.A., Kelsh, M.A., Lau, E.C., Edinboro, C.H., Barnard, J.C., Rutherford, G.W., Daaboul, J.J., Palmer, L., Lorey, F.W., "Thyroid function and perchlorate in drinking water: An evaluation among California newborns, 1998", Environmental Health Perspectives, 2006, 114(5), 798-804

181. Hooth, M.J., Deangelo, A.B., George, M.H., Gaillard, E.T., Travlos, G.S., Boorman, G.A., Wolf, D.C., "Subchronic sodium chlorate exposure in drinking water results in a concentration-dependent increase in rat thyroid follicular cell hyperplasia", Toxicologic Pathology, 2001, 29(2), 250-259

182. Flores, A., Hill, E.M., "Formation of estrogenic brominated ethinylestradiol in drinking water: implications for aquatic toxicity testing", Chemosphere, 2008, 73(7), 1115-1120

183. Jugan, M.L., Oziol, L., Bimbot, M., Huteau, V., Tamisier-Karolak, S.,

Blondeau, J.P., Levi, Y., "In vitro assessment of thyroid and estrogenic endocrine disrupters in wastewater treatment plants, rivers and drinking water supplies in the greater Paris area (France)", The Science of the Total Environment, 2009, 407(11), 3579-3587

184. Kuch, H.M., Ballschmiter, K., "Determination of endocrine-disrupting phenolic compounds and estrogens in surface and drinking water by HRGC-(NCI)-MS in the picogram per liter range", Environmental Science and Technology, 2001, 35(15), 3201-3206

185. Murr, A.S., Goldman, J.M., "Twenty-week exposures to the drinking water disinfection by-product dibromoacetic acid: reproductive cyclicity and steroid concentration in the female Sprague-Dawley rat", Reproductive Toxicology, 2005, 20(1), 73-80

186. Caldwell, D.J., Mastrocco, F., Nowak, E., Johnston, J., Yekel, H., Pfeiffer, D., Hoyt, M., DuPlessie, B.M., Anderson, P.D., "An assessment of potential exposure and risk from estrogens in drinking water", Environmental Health Perspectives, 2010, 118(3), 338-344

187. Falconer, I.R., "Are endocrine disrupting compounds a health risk in drinking water?" International Journal of Environmental Research and Public Health, 2006, 3(2), 180-184

188. Ward, M.H., deKok, T.M., Levallois, P., Brender, J., Gulis, G., Nolan, B.T., vanDerslice, J., "Workgroup report: Drinking-water nitrate and health - recent findings and research needs", Environmental Health Perspectives, 2005, 113, 1607-1614

189. Broberg, K., Concha, G., Engström, K., Lindvall, M., Grandér, M., Vahter, M., "Lithium in drinking water and thyroid function", Environmental Health Perspectives, 2011, 119(6), 827-830

190. Raymond-Whish, S., Mayer, L.P., O'Neal, T., Martinez, A., Sellers, M.A., Christian, P.J., Marion, S.L., Begay, C., Propper, C.R., Hoyer, P.B., Dyer, C.A., "Drinking water with uranium below the U.S. EPA water standard causes estrogen receptor-dependent responses in female mice", Environmental Health Perspectives, 2007, 115(12), 1711-1716

191. Buscemi, S., Mattina, A., Tranchina, M.R., Verga, S., "Acute effects of coffee on QT interval in healthy subjects", Nutrition Journal, 2011, 10 (15) Epub

192. Yoshida, Y., Hayakawa, M., Niki, E., "Evaluation of the antioxidant effects of coffee and its components using the biomarkers hydroxyoctadecadienoic acid and isoprostane", Journal of Oleo Science, 2008, 57(12), 691-697

193. Riemersma, R.A., Rice-Evans, C.A., Tyrrell, R.M., Clifford, M.N., Lean, M.E.J., "Tea flavonoids and cardiovascular health", QJM, 2001, 94, 277-282

194. Mustata, G.T., Rosca, M., Biemel, K.M., Reihl, O., Smith, M.A., Viswanathan, A., Strauch, C., Du, Y., Tang, J., Kern, T.S., Lederer, M.O., Brownlee, M., Weiss, M.F., Monnier, V.M., "Paradoxical effects of green tea (Camellia sinensis) and antioxidant vitamins in diabetic rats", Diabetes, 2005, 54, 517-526

195. Cabrera, C., Artacho, R., Giménez, R., "Beneficial effects of green tea - A review", Journal of the American College of Nutrition, 2006, 25(2), 79-99

196. Koo, S.I., Noh, S.K., "Green tea as inhibitor of the intestinal absorption of lipids: Potential mechanism for its lipid-lowering effect", Journal of Nutrition and Biochemistry, 2007, 18(3), 179-183

197. Zhong, L., Furne, J.K., Levitt, M.D., "An extract of black, green, and mulberry teas causes malabsorption of carbohydrate but not of triacylglycerol in health

volunteers", American Journal of Clinical Nutrition, 2006, 84, 551-555

198. Duffy, S.J., Vita, J.A., Holbrook, M., Swerdloff, P.L., Keaney, Jr., J.F., "Effect of acute and chronic tea consumption on platelet aggregation in patients with coronary artery disease", Arteriosclerosis, Thrombosis, and Vascular Biology, 2001, 21, 1084-1089

199. Negishi, H., Xu, J.-W., Ikeda, K., Njelekela, M., Nara, Y., Yamori, Y., "Black and green tea polyphenols attenuate blood pressure increases in stroke-prone spontaneously hypertensive rats", Journal of Nutrition, 2004, 134, 38-42

200. Duffy, S.J., Keaney Jr., J.F., Holbrook, M., Gokce, N., Swerdloff, P.L., Frei, B., Vita, J.A., "Short- and long-term black tea consumption reverses endothelial dysfunction in patients with coronary artery disease" Circulation, 2001, 104, 151-156

201. Henning, S.M., Niu, Y., Lee, N.H., Thames, G.D., Minutti, R.R., Wang, H., Go, V.L.W., Heber, D., "Bioavailability and antioxidant activity of tea flavanols after consumption of green tea, black tea, or a green tea extract supplement", American Journal of Clinical Nutrition, 2004, 80, 1558-1564

202. Hamden, K., Carreau, S., Marki, F.A., Masmoudi, H., El Feki, A., "Positive effects of green tea on hepatic dysfunction, lipid per oxidation and antioxidant defence depletion induced by cadmium", Biological Research, 2008, 41(3),331-339

203. Forester, S.C., Lambert, J.D., "The role of antioxidant versus pro-oxidant effects of green tea polyphenols in cancer prevention", Molecular Nutrition & Food Research, 2011, doi: 10.1002/mnfr.201000641

204. Abdeen, S.M., Mathew, T.C., Dashti, H.M., Asfar, S., "Protective effects of green tea on intestinal ischemia-reperfusion injury", Nutrition, 2011, 27(5), 598-603

205. Ribaldo, P.D.B., Souza, D.S., Biswas, S.K., Block, K., Lopes de Faria, J.M., Lopes de Faria, J.B., "Green tea (Camellia sinensis) attenuates nephropathy by downregulating Nox4 NADPH oxidase in diabetic spontaneously hypersensitive rats", The Journal of Nutrition, 2009, 139, 96-100

206. Lee, K.W., Lee, H.J., Lee, C.Y., "Antioxidant activity of black tea vs. green tea", Journal of Nutrition, 2002, 132, 785

207. Kurihara, H., Fukami, H., Asami, S., Toyoda, Y., Nakai, M., Shibata, H., Yao, X-S., "Effects of oolong tea on plasma antioxidative capacity in mice loaded with restraint stress assessed using the oxygen radical absorbance capacity (ORAC) assay", Biological & Pharmaceutical Bulletin, 2004, 27(7), 1093-1098

208. Shammas, M.A., Neri, P., Koley, H., Batchu, R.B., Bertheau, R.C., Munshi, V., Prabhala, R., Fulciniti, M., Tai, Y.T., Treon, S.P., Goyal, R.K., Anderson, K.C., Munshi, N.C., "Specific killing of multiple myeloma cells by (-)-epigallocatechin-3-gallate extracted from green tea: biologic activity and therapeutic implications", Blood, 2006, 108, 2804-2810

209. Nakazato, T., Ito, K., Ikeda, Y., Kizaki, M., "Green tea component, catechin, induces apoptosis of human malignant B cells via production of reactive oxygen species", Clinical Cancer Research, 2005, 11(16), 6040-6049

210. Mai, V., Katki, H.A., Harmsen, H., Gallaher, D., Schatzkin, A., Baer, D.J., Clevidence, B., "Effects of a controlled diet and black tea drinking on the fecal microflora composition and the fecal bile acid profile of human volunteers in a double-blinded randomized feeding study", Journal of Nutrition, 2004, 134, 473-478

211. Spencer, J.P.E., "Metabolism of tea flavonoids in the gastrointestinal tract", Proceedings of the Third International Scientific Symposium on Tea and Human Health: Role of Flavonoids in the Diet, The Journal of Nutrition, 2003, 133, 3255S-

3261S

212. Karmakar, S., Das, D., Maiti, A., Majumdar, S., Mukherjee, P., Das, A.S., Mitra, C., "Black tea prevents high fat diet-induced non-alcoholic steatohepatitis", Phytotherapy Research, 2011, March 31, 10.1002/ptr.3466 Epub

213. Chen, J.-H., Tipoe, G.L., Liong, E.C., So, H.S.H., Leung, K.-M., Tom, W.-M., Fung, P.C.W., Nanji, A.A., "Green tea polyphenols prevent toxin-induced hepatotoxicity in mice by down-regulating inducible nitric oxide-derived prooxidants", American Journal of Clinical Nutrition, 2004, 80, 742-751

214. Maxwell, S., Thorpe, G., "Tea flavonoids have little short term impact on serum antioxidant activity", British Medical Journal, 1996, 313, 229

215. López, V., Calvo, M.I., "White tea (Camellia sinensis Kuntze) exerts neuroprotection against hydrogen peroxide-induced toxicity in PC12 cells", Plant Foods for Human Nutrition, 2011, 66(11), 22-26

216. Kunishiro, K., Tai, A., Yamamoto, I., "Effects of rooibos tea extract on antigen-specific antibody production and cytokine generation in vitro and in vivo", Bioscience, Biotechnology and Biochemistry, 2001, 65(10), 2137-2145

217. Ulicna, O., Vancova, O., Bozek, P., Carsky, J., Sebekova, K., Boor, P., Nakano, M., Greksak, M., "Rooibos tea (Asphalathus linearis) partially prevents oxidative stress in streptozotocin-induced diabetic rats", Physiological Research, 2006, 55, 157-164

218. Kucharska, J., Ulicna, O., Gvozdjakova, A., Sumbalova, Z., Vancova, O., Bozek, P., Nakano, M., Greksak, M., "Regeneration of coenzyme Q9 redox state and inhibition of oxidative stress by rooibos tea (Aspalathus linearis) administration in carbon tetrachloride liver damage", Physiological Research, 2004, 53, 515-521

219. Liu, S.H., Chen, C., Yang, R.S., Yen, Y.P., Tsai, C., "Caffeine enhances osteoclast differentiation from bone marrow hematopoietic cells and reduces bone mineral density in growing rats", Journal of Orthopaedic Research, 2011, 29(6), 954-960

220. Zhou, Y., Guan, X.X., Zhu, Z.L., Guo, J., Huang, Y.C., Hou, W.W., Yu, H.Y., "Caffeine inhibits viability and osteogenic differentiation of rat bone marrow-derived mesenchymal stromal cells", British Journal of Pharmacology, 2010, 161(7), 1542-1552

221. Huang, T.H., Yang, R.S., Hsieh, S.S., Liu, S.H., "Effects of caffeine and exercise on the development of bone: a densitometric and histomorphometric study in young Wistar rats", Bone, 2002, 30(1), 293-299

222. Sakamoto, W., Nishihira, J., Fujie, K., Iizuka, T., Handa, H., Ozaki, M., Yukawa, S., "Effect of coffee consumption on bone metabolism", Bone, 2001, 28(3), 332-336

223. Dew, T.P., Day, A.J., Morgan, M.R., "Bone mineral density, polyphenols and caffeine: a reassessment", Nutrition Research Reviews, 2007, 20(1), 89-105

224. Heaney, R.P., "Effects of caffeine on bone and the calcium economy", Food and Chemical Toxicology, 2002, 40(9), 1263-1270

225. Ilich, J.Z., Brownhill, R.A., Tamborini, L., Crncevic-Orlic, Z., "To drink or not to drink: how are alcohol, caffeine and past smoking related to bone mineral density in elderly women?", Journal of the American Journal of Nutrition, 2002, 21(6), 536-544

226. Wetmore, C.M., Ichikawa, L., LaCroix, A.Z., Ott, S.M., Scholes, D., "Association between caffeine intake and bone mass among young women: potential effect modification by depot medroxyprogesterone acetate use", Osteoporosis International, 2008, 19(4), 519-527

227. Lloyd, T., Johnson Rollings, N., Kieselhorst, K., Eggli, D.F., Mauger, E., "Dietary caffeine intake is not correlated with adolescent bone gain", Journal of the American College of Nutrition, 1998, 17(5), 454-457

228. Lloyd, T., Johnson Rollings, N., Kieselhorst, K., Eggli, D.F., Mauger, E., Cusatis, D.C., "Bone status among postmenopausal women with different habitual caffeine intakes: A longitudinal study", Journal of the American College of Nutrition, 2000, 19(2), 256-261

229. Rapuri, P.B., Gallagher, J.C., Kinyamu, H.K., Ryschon, K.L., "Caffeine intake increases the rate of bone loss in elderly women and interacts with vitamin D receptor genotypes", American Journal of Clinical Nutrition, 2001, 74, 694-700

230. Hallström, H., Melhus, H., Glynn, A., Lind, L., Syvanen, A.-C., Michaelsson, K., "Coffee consumption and CYP1A2 genotype in relation to bone mineral density of the proximal femur in elderly men and women: a cohort study", Nutrition and Metabolism, 2010, 7(12) Epub

231. Goto, A., Song, Y., Chen, B.H., Manson, J.E., Buring, J.E., Liu, S., "Coffee and caffeine consumption in relation to sex hormone-binding globulin and risk of type 2 diabetes in postmenopausal women", Diabetes, 2011, 60(1), 269-275

232. Lopez-Garcia, E., Rodriguez-Artalejo, F., Rexrode, K.M., Logroscino, G., Hu, F.B., van Dam, R.M., "Coffee consumption and risk of stroke in women", Circulation, 2009, 119(8), 1116-1123

233. Pimental, G.D., Zemdegs, J.C.S., Theodoro, J.A., Mota, J.F., "Does long-term coffee intake reduce type 2 diabetes mellitus risk?", Diebetology & Metabolic Syndrome, 2009, 1(6) Epub

234. Lopez-Garcia, E., van Dam, R.M., Qui, L., Hu, F.B., "Coffee consumption and markers of inflammation and endothelial dysfunction in healthy and diabetic women", American Journal of Clinical Nutrition, 2006, 84, 888-893

235. Yu, X., Bao, Z., Zou, J., Dong, J., "Coffee consumption and risk of cancers: a meta-analysis of cohort studies", BMC Cancer, 2011, 11(96), Epub

236. Tverdal, A., Hjellvik, V., Selmer, R., "Coffee intake and oral-oesophageal cancer: follow-up of 389624 Norwegian men and women 40-45 years", British Journal of Cancer, 2011, 105, 157-161

237. Jernström, H., Henningson, M., Johansson, U., Olsson, H., "Coffee intake and CYP1A2*1F genotype predict breast volume in young women: implications for breast cancer", British Journal of Cancer, 2008, 99, 1534-1538

238. Durackova, Z., "Some current insights into oxidative stress", Physiological Research, 2010, 59, 459-469

239. Maiese, K., Chong, Z.Z., Hou, J., Shang, Y.C., "Oxidative stress: Biomarkers and novel therapeutic pathways", Experimental Gerontology, 2010, 45(3), 217-234

240. Bloomer, R.J., Kabir, M.M., Marshall, K.E., Canale, R.E., Farney, T.M., "Postprandial oxidative stress in response to dextrose and lipid meals of differing size", Lipids in Health and Disease, 2010, 9(79), Epub

241. Videla, L.A., "Oxidative stress signalling underlying liver disease and hepatoprotective mechanisms", World Journal of Hepatology, 2009, 1(1), 72-78

242. Kondo, T., Hirose, M., Kageyama, K., "Roles of oxidative stress and redox regulation in atherosclerosis", Journal of Atherosclerosis and Thrombosis, 2009, 16(5), 532-538

243. Armitage, M.E., Wingler, K., Schmidt, H.H.H.W., La, M., "Translating the oxidative stress hypothesis into the clinic: NOX versus NOS", Journal of Molecular

Medicine, 2009, 87, 1071-1076

244. Dotan, Y., Pinchuk, I., Lichtenburg, D., Leschno, M., "Decision analysis supports the paradigm that indiscriminate supplementation of vitamin E does more harm than good", Arteriosclerosis, Thrombosis, and Vascular Biology, 2009, 29, 1304-1309.

245. Marmol, F., Sanchez, J., Lopez, D., Martinez, N., Xuas, C., Peralta, C., Rosello-Catafau, J., Mitjavila, M.T., Puig-Parellada, P., "Role of oxidative stress and adenosine nucleotides in the liver of aging rats", Physiological Research, 2010, 59, 553-560

246. Duarte, T.L., Lunec, J., "When is an antioxidant not an antioxidant? A review of novel actions and reactions of vitamin C", Free Radical Research, 2005, 39, 671-686

247. Sharma, V., Anderson, D., Dhawan, A., "Zinc oxide nanoparticles induce oxidative stress and genotoxicity in human liver cells (HepG2)", Journal of Biomedical Nanotechnology, 2011, 7(1), 98-99

248. Sakurai, T., He, G., Matsuzawa, A., Yu, G.-Y., Maeda, S., Hardiman, G., Karin, M., "Hepatocyte necrosis induced by oxidative stress and IL-1alpha release mediate carcinogen-induced compensatory proliferation and liver tumorigenesis", Cancer Cell, 2008, 14(2), 156-165

249. Haces, M.L., Hernandez-Fonseca, K., Medina-Campos, O.N., Montiel, T., Pedraza-Chaverri, J., Massieu, L., "Antioxidant capacity contributes to protection of ketone bodies against oxidative damage induced during hypoglycaemic conditions", Experimental Neurology, 2008, 211, 85-96

250. Lisanti, M.P., Martinez-Outschoorn, U.E., Chiavarina, B., Pavlides, S., Whitaker-Menezes, D., Tsirigos, A., Witkiewicz, A., Lin, Z., Balliet, R., Howell, A., Sotgia, F., "Understanding the "lethal" drivers of tumor-stroma co-evolution: Emerging role(s) for hypoxia, oxidative stress and autophagy/mitophagy in the tumour micro-environment", Cancer Biology and Therapy, 2010, 10(6), 537-542

251. Abdelmegeed, M.A., Moon, K.H., Hardwick, J.P., Gonzalez, F.J., Song, B.J., "Role of peroxisome proliferator-activated receptor-alpha in fastring-mediated oxidative stress", Free Radical Biology and Medicine, 2009, 47(6), 767-778

252. Adams, S.D., Delano, B.A., Helmer, K.S., Mercer, D.W., "Fasting exacerbates and feeding diminishes LPS-induced liver injury in the rat", Digestive Diseases and Sciences, 2009, 54(4), 767-773

253. Sorensen, M., Sanz, A., Gomez, J., Pamplona, R., Portero-Otin, M., Gredilla, R., Barja, G., "Effects of fasting on oxidative stress in rat liver mitochondria", Free Radical Research, 2006, 40(4), 339-347

254. Salmi, H,., Hussain, K., Lapatto, R., "Change in plasma and erythrocyte thiol levels in children undergoing fasting studies for investigation of hypoglycaemia", Pediatric Endocrinology, Diabetes and Metabolism, 2011, 17(1), 14-19

255. Schindhelm, R.K., Alssema, M., Scheffer, P.G., Diamant, M., Dekker, J.M., Barto, R., Nijpels, G., Kostense, P.J., Heine, R.J., Schalkwijk, C.G., Teerlink, T., "Fasting and postprandial glycoxidative and lipoxidative stress are increased in women with type 2 diabetes", Diabetes Care, 2007, 30(7), 1789-1794

256. Wright Jr, E., Scism-Bacon, J.L., Glass, L.C., "Oxidative stress in type 2 diabetes: the role of fasting and postprandial glycaemia", International Journal of Clinical Practice, 2006, 60(3), 308-314

257. Svilaas, A., Sakhi, A.K., Andersen, L.F., Svilaas, T., Strom, E.C., Jacobs Jr., D.R., Ose, L., Blomhoff, R., "Intakes of antioxidants in coffee, wine, and vegetables are correlated with plasma carotenoids in humans", Journal of Nutrition, 2004, 134, 562-

567

258. Elizondo, A., Araya, J., Rodrigo, R., Signorini, C., Sgherri, C., Comporti, M., Poniachik, J., Videla, L.A., "Effects of weight loss on liver and erythrocyte polyunsaturated fatty acid pattern and oxidative stress status in obese patients with non-alcoholic fatty liver disease", Biological Research, 2008, 41(1), 59-68

259. Di Naso, F.C., Dias, A.S., Porawski, M., Marroni, N.A.P., "Exogenous superoxide dismutase: Action on liver oxidative stress in animals with streptozotocin-induced diabetes", Experimental Diabetes Research, 2011, doi:10.1155/2011/754132

260. Garcia-Compean, D., Jaquez-Quintana, J.O., Gonzalez-Gonzalez, J.A., Maldonado-Garza, H., "Liver cirrhosis and diabetes: Risk factors, pathophysiology, clinical implications and management", World Journal of Gastroenterology, 2009, 15(3), 280-288

261. Birch-Machin, M.A., Swalwell, H., "How mitochondria record the effects of UV exposure and oxidative stress using human skin as a model tissue", Mutagenesis, 2010, 25(2), 101-107

262. Roberts, R.A., Laskin, D.L., Smith, C.V., Robertson, F.M., Allen, E.M.G., Doorn, J.A., Slikker, W., "Nitrative and oxidative stress in toxicology and disease", Toxicological Sciences, 2009, 112(1), 4-16

263. Sugawara, T., Noshita, N., Lewen, A., Gasche, Y., Ferrand-Drake, M., Fukimura, M., Morita-Fujimura, Y., Chan, P.H., "Overexpression of copper-/zinc superoxide dismutase in transgenic rats protects vulnerable neurons against ischaemic damage by blocking the mitochondrial pathway of caspase activation", The Journal of Neuroscience, 2002, 22(1), 209-217

264. Vogiatzi, G., Tousoulis, D., Stefanadis, C., "The role of oxidative stress in atherosclerosis", Hellenic Journal of Cardiology, 2009, 50, 402-409

265. Aitkin, R.J., Roman, S.D., "Antioxidant systems and oxidative stress in the testes", Oxidative Medicine and Cellular Longevity, 2008, 1(1), 15-24

266. Ruder, E.H., Hartman, T.J., Goldman, M.B., "Impact of oxidative stress on female fertility", Current Opinions in Obstetrics and Gynecology, 2009, 21(3), 219-222

267. Beitz, R., Mensink, G.B., Hintzpeter, B., Fischer, B., Erbersdobler, H.F., "Do users of dietary supplements differ from nonusers in their food consumption?", European Journal of Epidemiology, 2004, 19(4), 335-341

268. Bolland, M.J., Grey, A., Avenell, A., Gamble, G.D., Reid, I.R., "Calcium supplements with or without vitamin D and risk of cardiovascular events: reanalysis of the Women's health initiative limited access database and meta-analysis", British Medical Journal, 2011; 342:d2040

269. Bolland, M.J., Grey, A., Reid, I.R., "Calcium supplements and cardiovascular risk", Journal of Bone and Mineral Research, 2011, January 4, Epub

270. Bolland, M.J., Avenell, A., Baron, J.A., Grey, A., MacLennan, G.S., Gamble, G.D., Reid, I.R., "Effect of calcium supplements on risk of myocardial infarction and cardiovascular events: meta-analysis", British Medical Journal, 2010, 341. doi:10.136/bmj.c3691

271. Lockwood, G.B., "The quality of commercially available nutraceutical supplements and food sources", Journal of Pharmacy and Pharmacology, 2011, 63(1), 3-10

272. Rehman, S., Adnan, M., Khalid, N., Shaheen, L., "Calcium supplements: an additional source of lead contamination", Biological Trace Element Research, 2010, October 15, Epub

273. Bourdon, J.A., Bazinet, T.M., Arnason, T.T., Kimpe, L.E., Blais, J.M., White, P.A., "Polychlorinated biphenyls (PCBs) contamination and aryl hydrocarbon receptor (AhR) agonist activity of omega-3 polyunsaturated fatty acid supplements: implications for daily intake of dioxins and PCBs", Food Chemistry and Toxicology, 2010, 48(11), 3093-3097

274. Petroczi, A., Taylor, G., Naughton, D.P., "Mission impossible? Regulatory and enforcement issues to ensure safety of dietary supplements", Food Chemistry and Toxicology, 2011, 49(2), 393-402

275. John, S.K., Rangan, Y., Block, C.A., Koff, M.D., "Life-threatening hyperkalemia from nutritional supplements: uncommon or undiagnosed?" American Journal of Emergency Medicine, 2010, November 12 (Epub)

276. Teschke, R., Schwarzenboeck, A., Hennermann, K.-H., "Causality assessment in hepatotoxicity by drugs and dietary supplements", British Journal of Clinical Pharmacology, 2008, 66(6), 758-766

277. Dara, L., Hewett, J., Lim, J.K., "Hydroxycut hepatotoxicity: A case series and review of liver toxicity from herbal weight loss supplements", World Journal of Gastroenterology, 2008, 14(45), 6999-7004

278. Chen, G.C., Ramanathan, V.S., Law, D., Funchain, P., Chen, G.C., French, S., Shlopov, B., Eysselein, V., Chung, D., Reicher, S., Pham, B.V., "Acute liver injury induced by weight-loss herbal supplements", World Journal of Hepatology, 2010, 2(11), 410-415

279. Stickel, F., Kessebohm, K., Weimann, R., Seitz, H.K., "Review of liver injury associated with dietary supplements", Liver International, 2011, 31(5), 595-605

280. Yellapu, R.K., Mittal, V., Grewal, P., Fiel, M., Schiano, T., "Acute liver failure caused by 'fat burners' and dietary supplements: a case report and literature review", Canadian Journal of Gastroenterology, 2011, 25(3), 157-160

281. Lobb, A., "Science of weight loss supplements: Compromised by conflicts of interest?", World Journal of Gastroenterology, 2010, 16(38), 4880-4882

282. Chan, J.M., Weinberg, V., Magbanua, M.J., Sosa, E., Simko, J., Shinokara, K., Federman, S., Mattie, M., Hughes-Fulford, M., Haqq, C., Carroll, P.R., "Nutritional supplements, COX-2 and IGF-1 expression in men on active surveillance for prostate cancer", Cancer Causes Control, 2011, 22, 141-150

283. Laidlow, M., Cockerline, C.A., Sepkovic, D.W., "Effects of a breast-health herbal formula supplement on estrogen metabolism in pre- and post-menopausal women not taking hormonal contraceptives or supplements: A randomised controlled trial", Breast Cancer: Basic and Clinical Research, 2010, 4, 85-95

284. Bjelakovic, G., Gluud, L.L., Nikolova, D., Bjelakovic, M., Nagorni, A., Gluud, C., "Antioxidant supplements for liver diseases", Cochrane Database Systematic Reviews, 2011, March 16, 3, CD007749

285. Liu, Q., Garner, P., Wang, Y., Huang, B., Smith, H., "Drugs and herbs given to prevent hepatotoxicity of tuberculosis therapy: systematic review of ingredients and evaluation studies", BMC Public Health, 2008, 8, 365, Epub

286. Rabovsky, A.B., Komarov, A.M., Ivie, J.S., Buettner, G.R., "Minimization of free radical damage by metal catalysis of multivitamin/multimineral supplements", Nutrition Journal, 2010, 9, 61, Epub

287. Yang, M., Chung, S.J., Chung, C.E., Kim, D.O., Song, W.O., Koo, S.I., Chun, O.K., "Estimation of total antioxidant capacity from diet and supplements in US adults", British Journal of Nutrition, 2011, Feb 15, 1-11

288. Heikkinen, A., Alaranta, A., Helenius, I., Vasankari, T., "Use of dietary supplements in Olympic athletes is decreasing: a follow-up study between 2002 and 2009", Journal of the International Society of Sports Nutrition, 2011, 8, 1, Epub

289. Lakhan, S.E., Vieira, K.F., "Nutritional and herbal supplements for anxiety and anxiety-related disorders: systematic review", Nutrition Journal, 2010, 9, 42, Epub

290. Norman, K., Pirlich, M., Smoliner, C., Kilbert, A., Schulzke, J.D., Ockenga, J., Lochs, H., Reinhold, T., "Cost-effectiveness of a 3-month intervention with oral nutritional supplements in disease-related malnutrition: a randomised controlled pilot study", European Journal of Clinical Nutrition, 2011, March 16, doi: 10.10138/ejcn.2011.31 Epub

291. Kawahito, S., Kitahata, H., Oshita, S., "Problems associated with glucose toxicity: Role of hyperglycaemia-induced oxidative stress", World Journal of Gastroenterology, 2009, 15(33), 4137-4142

292. Skinner, R., "Nephrotoxicity --what do we know and what don't we know?"Journal of Pediatric Hematology/Oncology, 2011, 33(2), 128-134

293. Cao, L.C., Honeyman, T.W., Cooney, R., Kennington, L., Scheid, C.R., Jonassen, J.A., "Mitochondrial dysfunction is a primary event in renal cell oxalate toxicity", Kidney International, 2004, 66(5), 1890-1900

294. Papa, S., Bubici, C., Zazzeroni, F., Franzoso, G., "Mechanisms of liver disease: The crosstalk between the NF-$_K$B and JNK pathways", Biological Chemistry, 2009, 390(10), 965-976

295. Mellion, M., Gilchrist, J.M., de la Monte, S., "Alcohol-induced peripheral neuropathy: nutritional, toxic, or both?", Muscle & Nerve, 2011, 43(3), 309-316

296. Brust, J.C.M., "Ethanol and cognition: Indirect effects, neurotoxicity and neuroprotection: A review", International Journal of Environmental Research and Public Health, 2010, 7, 1540-1557

297. Morleo, M., Woolfall, K., Dedman, D., Mukherjee, R., Bellis, M.A., Cook, P.A., "Under-reporting of foetal alchohol spectrum disorders: an analysis of hospital episode statistics", BMC Pediatrics, 2011, 11 (14) Epub

298. Stout, M.D., Herbert, R.A., Kissling, G.E., Suarez, F., Roycroft, J.H., Chhabra, R.S., Bucher, J.R., "Toxicity and carcinogenecity of methyl isobutyl ketone in F344N rats and B6C3F1 mice following two year inhalation exposure", Toxicology, 2008, 244(2-3), 209-219

299. Huang, S.W., Jin, J.Y., "Status of heavy metals in agricultural soils as affected by different patterns of land use", Environment Monitoring and Assessment, 2008, 139(1-3), 317-327

300. Yang, X.E., Long, X.X., Ni, W.Z., Ye, Z.Q., He, Z.L., Stoffella, P.J., Calvert, D.V., "Assessing copper thresholds for phytotoxicity and potential dietary toxicity in selected vegetable crops", Journal of Environmental Science and Health, Part B, 2002, 37(6), 625-635

301. Smith, E., Juhasz, A.L., Weber, J., "Arsenic uptake and speciation in vegetables grown under greenhouse conditions", Environmental Geochemistry and Health, 2009, 31(Supplement 1), 125-132

302. Wang, J., Fang, W., Yang, Z., Yuan, J., Zhu, Y., Yu, H., "Inter- and intraspecific variations of cadmium accumulation of 13 leafy vegetable species in a greenhouse experiment", Journal of Agriculture and Food Chemistry, 2007, 55(22), 9118-9123

303. LoPachin, R.M., Barber, D.S., Geohagen, B.C., Gavin, T., He, D., Das, S.,

References

"Structure-toxicity analysis of Type-2 alkenes: In vitro neurotoxicity", Toxicology Sciences, 2007, 95(1), 136-146

304. Summerfield, W., Goodson, A., Cooper, I., "Survey of bisphenol a diglycidyl ether (BADGE) in canned foods", Food Additives and Contaminants, 1998, 15(7), 818-830

305. Dionisi, G., Oldring, P.K., Joint Industry Group (JIG), "Estimates of per capita exposure to substances migrating from canned foods and beverages", Food Additives and Contaminants, 2002, 19(9), 891-903

306. Misra, U.K., Kalita, J., "Toxic neuropathies", Neurology India, 2009, 57(6), 697-705

307. Morgan, D.L., Price, H.C., O'Conner, R.W., Seely, J.C., Ward, S.M., Wilson, R.E., Cunningham, M.C., "Upper respiratory tract toxicity of inhaled methylvinyl ketone in F344 rats and B6C3F1 mice", Toxicology Sciences, 2000, 58, 182-194

308. Thrash, B., Thiruchelvan, K., Ahuja, M., Suppiramaniam, V., Dhanasekaran, M., "Methamphetamine-induced neurotoxicity: the road to Parkinson's disease", Pharmacological Reports, 2009, 61, 966-977

309. Perouansky, M., Hemmings, H.C., "Neurotoxicity of general anesthetics: Cause for concern?", Anesthesiology, 2009, 111(6), 1365-1371

310. Arteel, G.E., "Alcohol-induced oxidative stress in the liver", Methods in Molecular Biology, 2008, 447, 185-197

311. Velchik, M.G., Reynolds, J.C., Alavi, A., "The effect of meal energy content on gastric emptying", Journal of Nuclear Medicine, 1989, 30, 1106-1110

312. Hunt, J.N., Stubbs, D.F., "The volume and energy content of meals as determinants of gastric emptying", Journal of Physiology, 1975, 245, 209-225

313. Clegg, M., Shafat, A., "Energy and macronutrient composition of breakfast affect gastric emptying of lunch and subsequent food intake, satiety and satiation", Appetite, 2010, 54(3), 517-523

314. Göranzon, H., Forsum, E., Thilen, M., "Calculation and determination of metabolizable energy in mixed diets to humans", The American Journal of Clinical Nutrition, 1983, 38, 954-963

315. Jumpertz, R., Le, D.S., Turnbaugh, P.J., Trinidad, C., Bogardus, C., Gordon, J.I., Krakoff, J., "Energy-balance studies reveal associations between gut microbes, caloric load, and nutrient absorption in humans", American Journal of Clinical Nutrition, 2011, May 4, epub

316. Miles, C.W., "The metabolizable energy of diets differing in dietary fat and fiber measured in humans", The Journal of Nutrition, 1992, 122, 306-311

317. Baile, C.A., Della-Fera, M.A., Martin, R.J., "Regulation of metabolism and body fat mass by leptin", Annual Review of Nutrition, 2000, 20, 105-127

318. Foltin, R.W., Rolls, B.J., Moran, T.H., Kelly, T.H., McNelis, A.L., Fischman, M.W., "Caloric, but not macronutrient, compensation by humans for required-eating occasions with meals and snack varying in fat and carbohydrate", American Journal of Clinical Nutrition, 1992, 55, 331,342

319. Wansink, B., Chandon, P., "Meal size, not body size, explains errors in estimating the calorie content of meals", Annals of Internal Medicine, 2006, 145(5), 326-332

320. Speakman, J.R., Walker, H., Walker, L., Jackson, D.M., "Associations between BMI, social strata and the estimated energy content of foods", International Journal of Obesity (London), 2005, 29(10), 1281-1288

321. Yeomans, M.R., Lartamo, S., Procter, E.L., Lee, M.D., Gray, R.W., "The actual, but not labelled, fat content of a soup preload alters short-term appetite in healthy men", Physiology & Behaviour, 2001, 73(4), 533-540

322. Smith, S.R., de Jonge, L., Zachwieja, J.J., Roy, H., Nguyen, T., Rood, J., Windhauser, M., Volaufova, J., Bray, G.A., "Concurrent physical activity increases fat oxidation during the shift to a high-fat diet", American Journal of Clinical Nutrition, 2000, 72, 131-138

323. Westerterp, K.R., "Diet induced thermogenesis", Nutrition & Metabolism, 2004, 1(5), Epub

324. Kinabo, J.L., Durnin, J.V., "Thermic effect of food in man: effect of meal compensation, and energy content", British Journal of Nutrition, 1990, 64(1), 37-44

325. Blaak, E.E., Hul, G., Verdich, C., Stich, V., Martinez, J.A., Petersen, M., Feskins, E.F.M., Patel, K., Oppert, J.M., Barbe, P., Toubro, S., Polak, J., Anderson, I., Astrup, A., Macdonald, I., Langin, D., Sorensen, T., Saris, W.H., NUGENOB Consortium, "Impaired fat-induced thermogenesis in obese: The NUGENOB study", Obesity, 2007, 15(3), 653-663

326. Nowson, C.A., Patchett, A., Wattanapenpaiboon, N., "The effects of a low-sodium base-producing diet including red meat compared with a high-carbohydrate, low-fat diet on bone turnover markers in women aged 45-75 years", British Journal of Nutrition, 2009, 102(8), 1161-1170

327. Lam, T.K., Cross, A.J., Consonni, D., Randi, G., Bagnardi, V., Bertazzi, P.A., Caporaso, N.E., Sinha, R., Subar, A.F., Landi, M.T., "Intakes of red meat, processed meat, and meat mutagens increase lung cancer risk", Cancer Research, 2009, 69(3), 932-939

328. Dyall, S.C., Michael, G.J., Whelpton, R., Scott, A.G., Michael-Titus, A.T., "Dietary enrichment with omega-3 polyunsaturated fatty acids reverses age-related decreases in the GluR2 and NR2B glutamate receptor subunits in rat forebrain", Neurobiology of Aging, 2007, 28(3), 424-439

329. Dyall, S.C., Michael, G.J., Michael-Titus, A.T., "Omega-3 fatty acids reverse age-related decreases in nuclear receptors and increase neurogenesis in old rats", Journal of Neuroscience Research, 2010, 88(10), 2091-2102

330. Simopoulos, A.P., "The importance of omega-6/omega-3 fatty acid ratio in cardiovascular disease and other chronic diseases", Experimental Biology and Medicine, 2008, 233(6), 674-688

331. Simopoulos, A.P., "Importance of omega-6/omega-3 balance in health and disease: evolutionary aspects of diet", World Review of Nutrition and Dietetics, 2011, 102, 10-21

332. Grieger, J.A., Nowson, C.A., "Use of calcium, folate, and vitamin D-fortified milk for 6 months improves nutritional status but not bone mass or turnover, in a group of Australian aged care residents", Journal of Nutrition for the Elderly, 2009, 28(3), 236-254

333. Kanis, J.A., Johansson, H., Oden, A., De Laet, C., Johnell, O., Eisman, J.A., McClockey, E., Mellstrom, D., Pols, H., Reeve, J., Silman, A., Tenenhouse, A., "A meta-analysis of milk intake and fracture risk: low utility for case finding", Osteoporosis International, 2005, 16(7), 799-804

334. Fransen, H.P., Pelgrom, M.G.J., Stewart-Knox, B., de Kaste, D., Verhagen, H., "Assessment of health claims, content, and safety of herbal supplements containing

References

Gingko biloba", Food and Nutrition Research, 2010, 54, 5221 - DOI: 10.3402/fnrv54i0.5221

335. Jeon, Y.J., Myung, S.K., Lee, E.H., Kim, Y., Chang, Y.J., Ju, W., Cho, H.J., Seo, H.G, Huh, B.Y., "Effects of beta-carotene supplements on cancer prevention: meta-analysis of randomised controlled trials", Nutrition and Cancer, 2011, October 7 (Epub).

336. Lee, E.H., Myung, S.K., Jeon, Y.J., Kim, Y., Chang, Y.J., Ju, W., Seo, H.G., Huh, B.Y., "Effects of selenium supplements on cancer prevention: Meta-analysis of randomised controlled trials", Nutrition and Cancer, 2011, October 17 (Epub).

337. Bischoff-Ferrari, H.A., Dawson-Hughes, B., Baron, J.A., Kanis, J.A., Orav, E.J., Staehelin, H.B., Kiel, D.P., Burckhardt, P., Henschkowski, J., Spiegelman, D., Li, R., Wong, J.B., Feskanich, D., Willett, W.C., "Milk intake and risk of hip fracture in men and women: A meta-analysis of prospective cohort studies", Journal of Bone and Mineral Research, 2011, 26(4), 833-839

338. Bobulescu, I.A., Moe, O.W., "Na^+/H^+ exchangers in renal regulation of acid-base balance", Seminars in Nephrology, 2006, 26(5), 334-344

339. Davies, M.J., Judd, J.T., Baer, D.J., Clevidence, B.A., Paul, D.R., Edwards, A.J., Wiseman, S.A., Muesing, R.A., Chen, S.C., "Black tea consumption reduced total and LDL cholesterol in mildly hypercholesterolemic adults", Proceedings of the Third International Scientific Symposium on Tea and Human Health: Role of Flavonoids in the Diet, Journal of Nutrition, 2003, 133, 3298S-3302S

340. Larsson, S.C., Mannisto, S., Virtanen, M.J., Kontto, J., Albanes, D., Virtamo, J., "Dairy foods and risk of stroke", Epidemiology, 2009, 20(3), 355-360